CONSULTANTS FOR THIS BOOK

Jack H. Wilmore, Ph.D., is the Margie Gurley Seay Centennial Professor in the Department of Education at the University of Texas at Austin. He is a Fellow of the American College of Sports Medicine, the author of *Athletic Training and Physical Fitness: Principles and Practices of the Conditioning Process* and *The Wilmore Fitness Program*. He is co-author of *Evaluation and Regulation of Body Build and Composition* and editor of *Exercise and Sports Sciences Review*.

Risa Friedman, M.A., is Program Director of the Fitness Specialist Certification Program at Marymount Manhattan College in New York City. Certified by the American College of Sports Medicine, the International Dance Exercise Association and The Laban-Bartenieff Institute, Friedman has taught anatomy/kinesiology, movement analysis, therapeutic exercise, exercise physiology, and fitness and dance at New York University and Skidmore College, among other institutions.

Myron Winick, M.D., is the R.R. Williams Professor of Nutrition, Professor of Pediatrics, Director of the Institute of Human Nutrition, and Director of the Center for Nutrition, Genetics and Human Development at Columbia University College of Physicians and Surgeons. He has served on the Food and Nutrition Board of the National Academy of Sciences and is the author of many books, including *Your Personalized Health Profile*.

For information about any Time-Life book please write:
Reader Information
Time-Life Books
541 North Fairbanks Court
Chicago
Illinois 60611

Library of Congress Cataloging-in-Publication Data
Getting firm.
Includes index.
1. Physical fitness. 2. Exercise. 3. Nutrition.
I. Time-Life Books.
GV481.G47 1987 613.7'1 86-30000
ISBN 0-8094-6158-7
ISBN 0-8094-6159-5 (lib. bdg.)

This book is not intended as a substitute for the advice of a physician. Readers who have, or suspect they may have, specific medical problems, especially those involving their muscles and joints, are urged to consult a physician before beginning any program of strenuous physical exercise.

CONTENTS

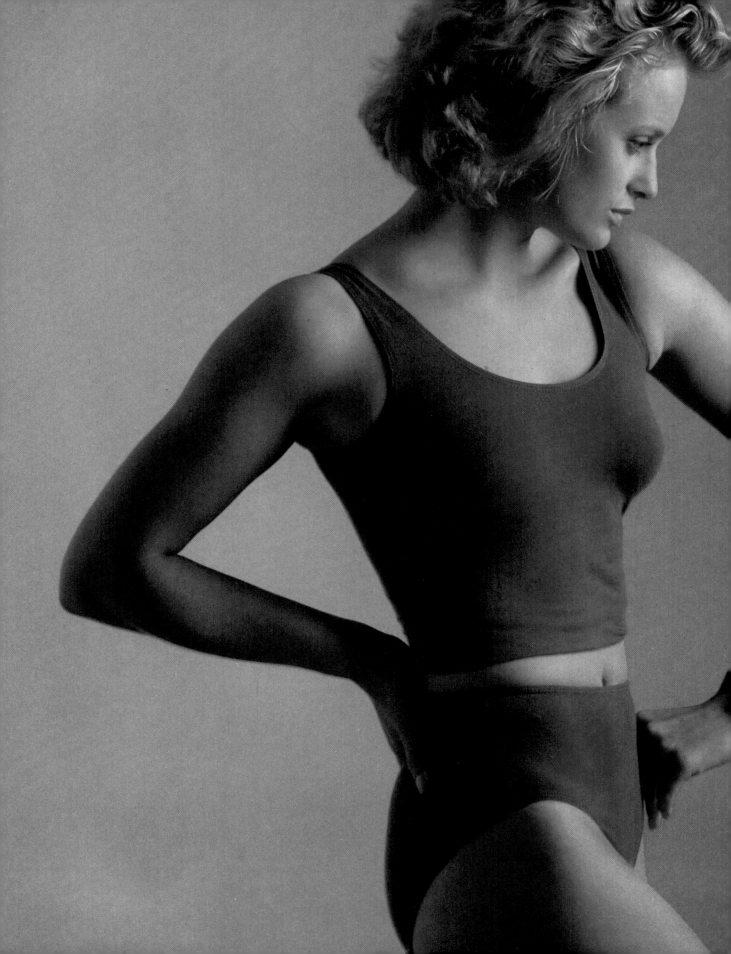

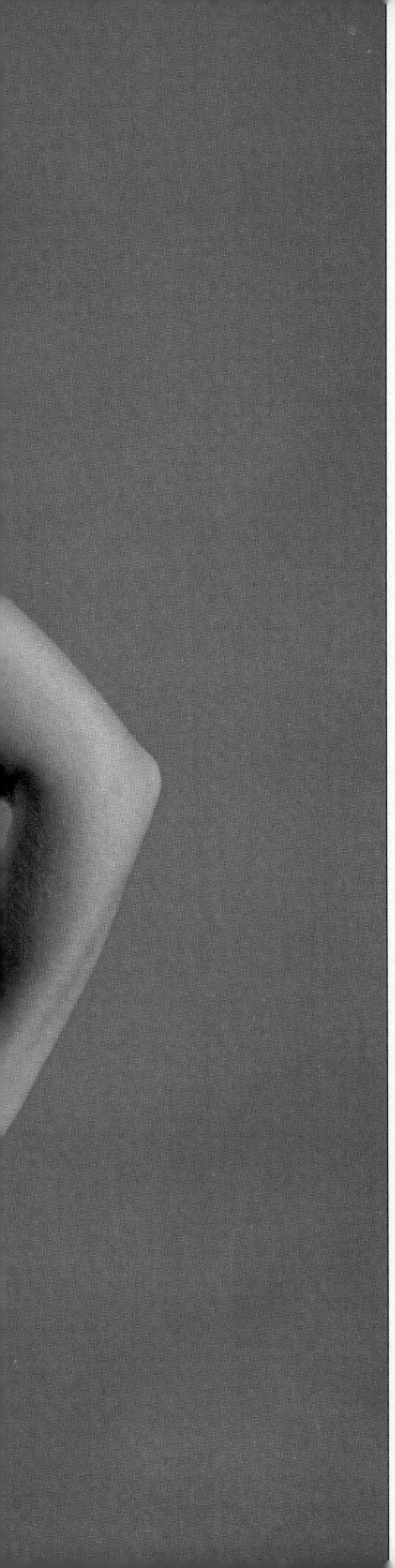

CHAPTER ONE

Shaping and Toning

*Toward firmer muscles
and a more impressive
physique — with the dividend
of added strength*

Y ou cannot grow new muscles, any more than you can add inches to your height or alter your basic body type. But you can change the tone and shape of your muscles, whatever your body type, and so bridge the gap between the physique you want and the one confronting you in the mirror every day.

The muscles that shape our physiques are skeletal muscles, and there are more than 400 of them. (The other 200 muscles of the body are not affected by shaping and toning exercises. These muscles include the cardiac muscle and the smooth muscles that perform such functions as moving food through the digestive tract and constricting blood vessels to regulate blood flow.) Many people assume that to get firm requires dozens of exercises. The truth is, you do not need a lot of exercises — a few very basic ones, done correctly, will take you a long way toward your goal.

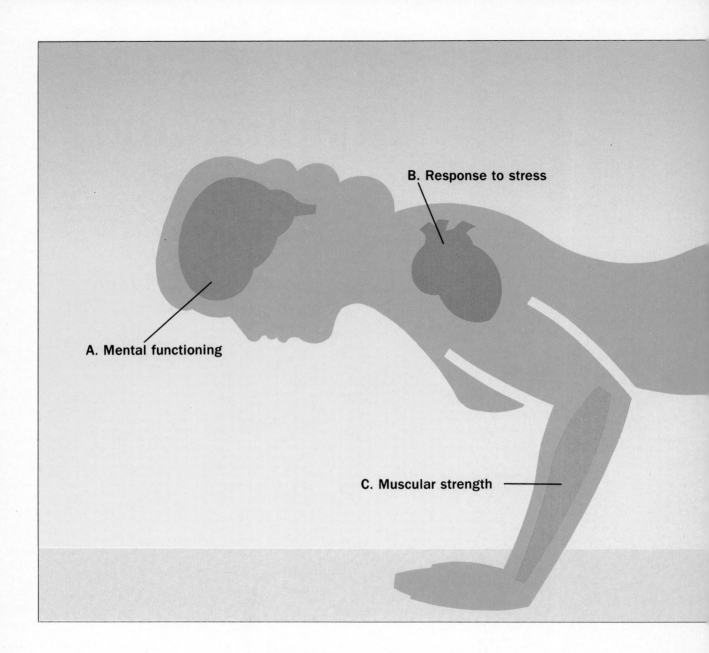

B. Response to stress

A. Mental functioning

C. Muscular strength

What exactly is muscle tone?

In a technical sense, muscle tone is a state of residual tension — that is, a muscle being contracted even at rest. Researchers have discovered, however, that only smooth muscles, like those of the intestinal wall, maintain such a long-term, steady contraction (which is also called "tonus"). The skeletal muscles — the ones you shape and strengthen — may not contract at all when they are at rest. What we call muscle tone is not the contraction of your muscles, but rather their appearance and health. Toned muscles look and feel resilient: They do not droop at the back of the arm or sag at the waist. If you perform the exercises in this book, you will find that your muscles become shapelier and firmer to the touch, whether you are working out or standing still.

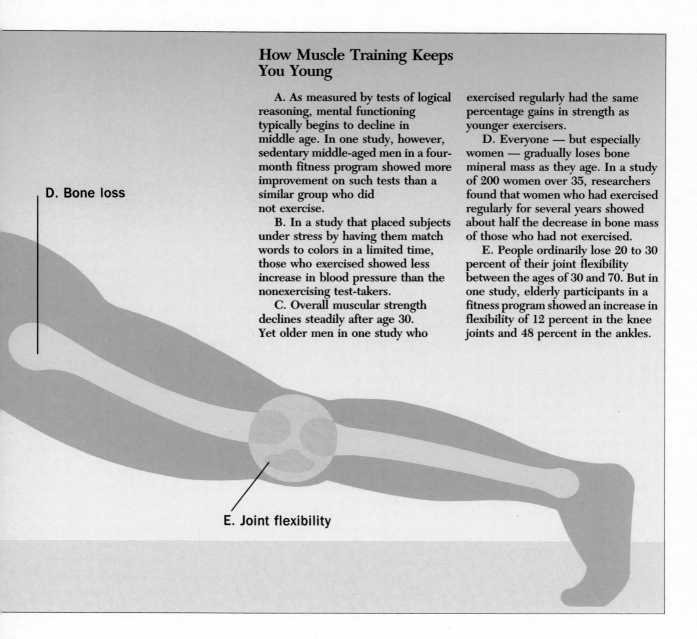

How Muscle Training Keeps You Young

A. As measured by tests of logical reasoning, mental functioning typically begins to decline in middle age. In one study, however, sedentary middle-aged men in a four-month fitness program showed more improvement on such tests than a similar group who did not exercise.

B. In a study that placed subjects under stress by having them match words to colors in a limited time, those who exercised showed less increase in blood pressure than the nonexercising test-takers.

C. Overall muscular strength declines steadily after age 30. Yet older men in one study who exercised regularly had the same percentage gains in strength as younger exercisers.

D. Everyone — but especially women — gradually loses bone mineral mass as they age. In a study of 200 women over 35, researchers found that women who had exercised regularly for several years showed about half the decrease in bone mass of those who had not exercised.

E. People ordinarily lose 20 to 30 percent of their joint flexibility between the ages of 30 and 70. But in one study, elderly participants in a fitness program showed an increase in flexibility of 12 percent in the knee joints and 48 percent in the ankles.

D. Bone loss

E. Joint flexibility

What good will shaping and toning do you?

The most obvious reward of a shaping and toning program is a pleasingly contoured body. But when you tone muscles, you also strengthen them — in terms of both absolute strength (the ability to lift a weight once) and muscular endurance (the ability to repeat a muscular contraction many times in quick succession). Endurance allows muscles to make a sustained effort, which in your day-to-day life will mean a greater resistance to fatigue. And firm muscles reinforce the joints they support, so that you are less likely to stress or strain a knee, ankle or elbow.

Furthermore, skeletal muscles support the more than 200 bones that make up the body. If muscles are not sufficiently firm, bones do not handle the load properly. The result: Shoulders slump, the back humps, the neck slopes forward. This poor posture not only looks unattractive, but puts pressure on nerves and disks along the spine, often producing back pain as well as pain or numbness in the extremities. When you exercise back-related muscles, you help keep the spine aligned and take pressure off vulnerable areas of the lower back.

Fat vs. Muscle

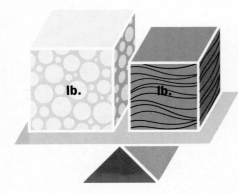

A pound of fat takes up about 20 percent more room than a pound of muscle. But a pound of muscle burns more calories, even at rest, than fat does. Moreover, excessive body fat places an added burden on your heart, lungs, kidneys and liver without giving anything in return.

If muscle-toning exercises provide muscular endurance, do they also give you aerobic endurance?
Any muscle that contracts repeatedly for more than two minutes requires fresh oxygen and is therefore drawing on energy that is aerobic, meaning "with air." But the common meaning of aerobic endurance is the ability of the heart, lungs and blood vessels — your cardiovascular system — to deliver ever-larger amounts of oxygen to working muscles during activities like running, brisk walking, swimming or cycling. To build up your cardiovascular system, you need to sustain such activities at a vigorous pace for at least 20 minutes. Fast-paced muscle-toning exercises may accelerate your heartbeat substantially, but only the specific muscles worked receive the benefit of muscular endurance. The body's handling of oxygen (cardiovascular endurance) does not get a workout.

Isn't an activity like swimming, which works the whole body, really better for getting firm?
Swimming is a superb exercise, but you cannot use it to target specific muscles for development, as you can with the exercises in this book. And you can do these shaping and toning exercises conveniently at home, away from the pool or beach.

But do you really need to be shown how to do sit-ups and push-ups?
Yes. For one thing, the conventional sit-up is dangerous. Keeping your legs flat on the floor arches the lower back, which overextends it and places it under stress. Then, too, sitting up fully during a sit-up — instead of just lifting your head and shoulders up off the floor — brings your hip-flexor muscles into play, arching the lower back again and placing it under stress. Finally, putting your hands behind your head and jerking up to get yourself started on a sit-up places a potentially damaging stress on your neck. Push-ups do not pose such hazards, but the proper techniques and several variations are crucial to getting the most from your workout.

How much do you need to work out?
For the exercises in this book to have any benefit, you need to do them at least three times a week. If you are out of shape, you can exercise all of your major muscle groups in about 30 minutes. But if you have been doing an exercise like running, swimming or aerobic movement, some of your muscles may already be firm, allowing you to shorten your shaping and toning workouts. The most important fact to

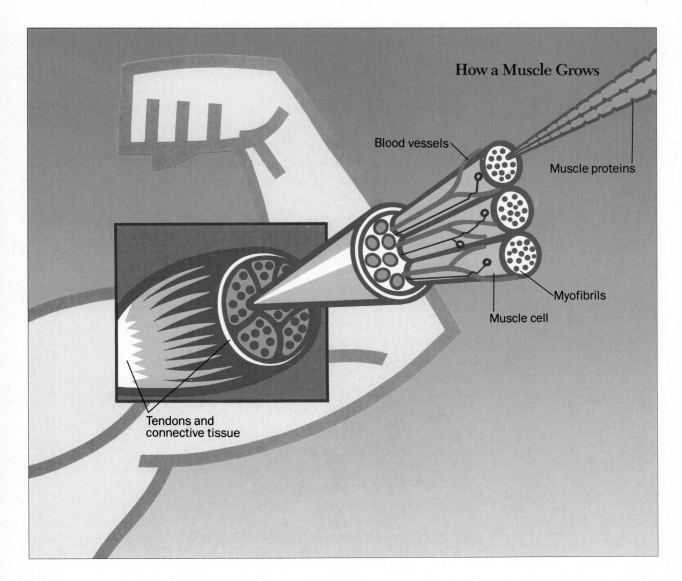

How a Muscle Grows

Blood vessels

Muscle proteins

Myofibrils

Muscle cell

Tendons and
connective tissue

remember is that you should balance your workouts with recuperation time. Many people choose not to work the same muscle groups two days in a row. You can, if you wish, do the same exercises five or six days a week once you have worked up to it. But give yourself at least one day off a week.

How hard should you work out?

For advice on how to design a program for yourself, see pages 16-17. As a rule, however, you should work enough to feel the effort. If you are completely comfortable in a workout, you are not working hard enough. If you begin to feel pain, you have gone too far and should stop exercising at once.

What is the best time to work out?

Your body is ordinarily warmest and most relaxed in the evening, which makes that the best time to work out. But any time is good

When a muscle is exercised repeatedly and vigorously for an extended period, it grows larger. Most experts agree that this growth takes place because the cells that make up the muscle, and the structures that contain and support the cells, increase in size and strength. (The number of cells, also called muscle fibers, remains the same.) The tendons and connective tissue surrounding the muscle increase in size, and the blood vessels expand and proliferate. Inside each muscle cell, more myofibrils — the structures that contract — are created, as are the muscle proteins (such as myosin) that compose them.

11

except for the first 20 minutes after you wake up in the morning, when your body has not yet warmed up.

Is there any proven way to boost your motivation so that you stay with an exercise program?
There certainly is. Many studies have shown that people stay with programs when they exercise with a spouse or a friend. If you do work out with a partner, however, remember that these workouts are not a competitive sport: Do not overextend yourself just to keep up with your exercise partner.

How soon will you see results?
You should see a change in four weeks.

To what extent is good muscle tone inherited?
The extent to which you can shape your muscles is partly genetic. Mesomorphs, with their muscular, V-shaped bodies, have an easier time acquiring and keeping muscle tissue than either ectomorphs (slender bodies) or endomorphs (plump bodies). Within these limits, however, you can dramatically improve the appearance of your muscles by getting rid of the body fat that obscures them and by performing the exercises in this book.

Will these exercises give you bulging muscles?
They will give you taut muscles, not bulging ones. The only way you can build bulging muscles is with weight training, but even that will not necessarily make you bulky. The entrants in body-building contests acquire much of their potential for muscle bulk from their genes. They also work out daily, lifting weights in strenuous routines until their muscles are exhausted. Working with lighter weights to bring your muscles to a size and shape that appeal to you will not make you look like a body builder. The exercises in this book are designed to tone you, not build you up.

If you stop exercising, will the muscle turn to fat?
No. Muscle and fat are two entirely different, highly specialized tissues that are incapable of turning into one another. But exercise and its opposite, inactivity, can alter the distribution and mass of muscle and fat in ways that create the illusion that a transformation is taking place.

If you exercise your arm and leg muscles, for instance, they will grow larger. To maintain these better-toned muscles, your body will use more calories, eventually drawing on the fat stored in layers of tissue beneath the skin and over the muscles — not just from those areas where you have toned your muscles, but from all over the body. As the deposits of fat decline, the contours of the arm and leg muscles will become increasingly visible.

If you do not use your muscles, however, they will gradually shrink.

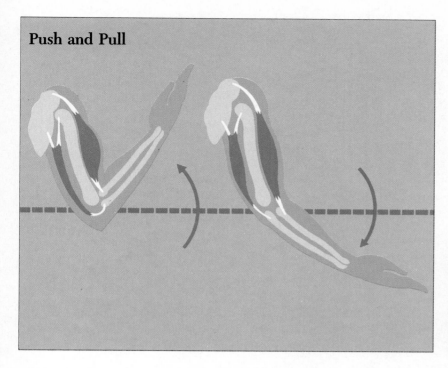

Push and Pull

Muscles can only pull; they cannot push. Therefore, muscles always act in pairs to move your body: The arm shown at left moves upward when the biceps contracts and thickens, while the triceps relaxes. When the arm is forcibly extended, the triceps contracts. Because of this arrangement, you must always work two opposing muscles in order to shape and tone any part of your body completely.

At the same time, any calories you consume in excess of those you burn up for energy will be banked as fat, with a good share of them deposited directly over your muscles.

Do strength-building exercises make you less flexible?
Not at all. As a matter of fact, strength training can make you more flexible, not less, since any exercise that takes your muscles through their full range of motion stretches them. Most of the exercises in this book require a particular part of your body to be moved through its full range — thus enhancing flexibility.

What if you have back trouble? Will these exercises help?
Anyone with back trouble should see a doctor before doing exercises. If you do not have back problems, you should do some exercises to help you avoid them. One of the most important things you can do is to strengthen your abdominal muscles. When these muscles are strong, they help bring your posture into proper alignment, which is a key to supporting the back. In general, the stronger you are, the less prone you are to injury. Of course, if any exercise causes back pain, stop doing it immediately.

Can you use these exercises to get rid of fat around your waist or on your thighs?
No. You cannot "spot reduce." The best way to reduce is to cut your caloric intake and burn calories by sustained aerobic exercise, which will gradually reduce fat all over. Since women store a good deal of fat

13

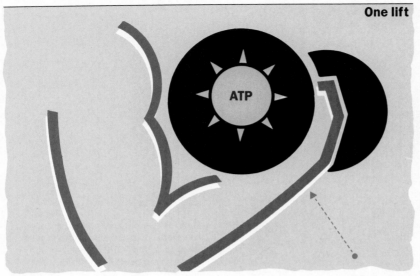

One lift

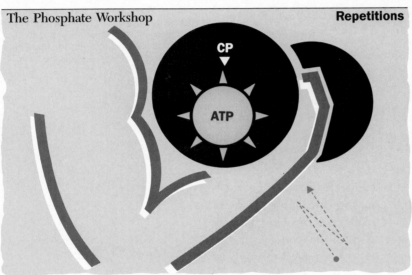

The Phosphate Workshop

Repetitions

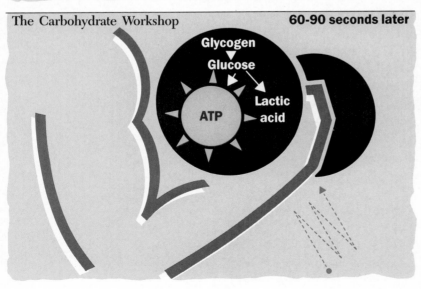

The Carbohydrate Workshop

60-90 seconds later

Quick Energy for Building Muscles

The energy you use to shape and strengthen muscles is different from the energy you draw on to give them endurance. In fact, you make a muscle stronger by tiring it. When you lift a weight — or lift your own body weight by doing a push-up or chin-up — the muscle instantly taps a limited reserve of adenosine triphosphate, or ATP, the fuel that powers all muscular contractions. The muscle expends its entire store of ATP in a second or two and must then manufacture more.

As the muscle continues lifting the weight, it synthesizes more ATP from a small supply of another stored substance called creatine phosphate, or CP. The CP will drive the muscle for another eight to 10 seconds; then it, too, is used up.

If the exercise continues, the muscle depletes all of its phosphate reserves and turns to carbohydrates to generate ATP anaerobically, or "without oxygen." This involves converting glycogen stored in the muscle into glucose — a process that produces ATP and a by-product called lactic acid. Anaerobic energy can power the muscle for 60 to 90 seconds, depending on the size of the muscle and the intensity of the exercise. As the lactic acid builds up, it causes the muscle to fatigue.

By that point, the effort of lifting the weight has engaged as many muscle fibers as possible. If you reduce your level of exertion, your muscle will produce longer-lasting aerobic energy to continue contracting. But for further gains in muscle tone and strength, which require a relatively short, intense effort, the muscle must rest before going to work again.

in their lower bodies, they will notice that aerobic exercise has taken off some of that fat. Since men store most of their fat around their waists and in their upper bodies, they will experience fat loss in those areas.

Will it help you reduce if you wear a rubber or vinyl exercise suit?
You will experience only a temporary water-weight loss, which may be dangerous. Such a suit causes your body to heat up by stalling your normal cooling mechanism, which is the evaporation of perspiration. So your body perspires, your fluid reserves go down and your temperature goes up. You can suffer serious dehydration — conceivably even death from heatstroke — when you exercise under these conditions.

Will a steam bath or sauna tone you as well as exercises?
You may feel toned and trimmed after a steam bath or sauna because you have lost weight, but the weight you have lost is all water and salt, which you will quickly regain. As a method of losing weight and toning, sitting in a sauna or steam room is no better than sitting at a desk or in your living room.

What is the best way to get a flat stomach?
You need to do aerobic exercises to burn off fat and the crunches on pages 60-66 to firm up the muscles underneath.

Is it true you might look trimmer but actually weigh more?
Yes. Muscle is denser than fat, so if you lose fat tissue but add muscle, your weight may climb. But you will probably look like you have lost weight, since muscles are firmer and more pleasing to the eye than fat, and, even though your weight may go up, your waistline may actually shrink. Furthermore, most people will not gain more than two or three pounds of muscle from body-shaping workouts.

Will eating a lot of protein, especially red meat, make muscles firmer or stronger?
Exercise, not protein or protein supplements, improves your strength, power and endurance. Not even body builders need more protein in their diets than the average person already eats. In all likelihood, body builders consume more protein than they need, perhaps two to three times more. A 150-pound man needs about 55 grams of protein in his diet every day; a 120-pound woman, about 44 grams. Half a cup of cottage cheese will give you 14 grams. A four-ounce piece of chicken will give you 31 grams. An eight-ounce cup of milk will give you 8.5 grams. It is not hard to get enough protein; chances are you already eat too much. What is hard is to get protein without consuming a lot of fat. *(For some recipes that deal with this problem, see pages 128-141.)*

How to Design Your Own Program

Most of us do not need laboratory tests to confirm that we are in good or bad shape. A look in the mirror tells us all we want to know — and sometimes a lot more. And we can tell how our bodies feel to us, whether we are sedentary or active. But, to begin to think a bit more analytically about such matters, we might want to consider the questions to the right.

Are you in good shape?

1 Do you end the day with reserves of strength?

Fitness, according to the President's Council on Physical Fitness, is "the ability to carry out daily tasks with vigor and alertness, without undue fatigue and with ample energy to enjoy leisure-time pursuits and to meet unforeseen emergencies." To be sure, much of the feeling of vigor that this definition mentions must come from aerobic activities such as running, swimming or cycling. But the strength to heft a suitcase, to add force to your golf swing or your tennis serve, or simply to sit or stand comfortably for long periods comes from the kind of exercises that are in this book.

2 Are you small-boned? Fair-skinned? Female?

Both men and women suffer some bone loss as they get older, but a dangerous weakening of the bones (osteoporosis) afflicts fully 25 percent of all women over the age of 65 — a weakening that begins early and increases dramatically with menopause. Women typically lose 30 percent of their bone mass between the ages of 30 and 70. Being small-boned or fair-skinned, smoking, dieting often, being underweight most of your life, exercising infrequently and not consuming enough calcium are all associated with a high risk of osteoporosis. To make up for a calcium deficiency, your body must take calcium out of the bones and use it for vital functions. Deprived of much of their calcium, bones become weak and vulnerable to fractures.

Some women find it advisable to take calcium supplements or eat calcium-rich foods after the age of 35. But a study done at the Biogerontology Laboratory at the University of Wisconsin demonstrated conclusively that exercise is a superb bone strengthener. The Wisconsin study put a number of older women (average age: 84) through a program of gentle toe taps, arm lifts, sideways bends and slow knee lifts in 30-minute sessions three times a week. The exercise not only stemmed bone loss, but actually stimulated the bones to produce new cells. Mechanical stress on the bones stimulates the growth of cells called osteoblasts. The increase in bone formation is directly proportional to the amount of stress applied.

While the problem of bone loss is particularly acute for women, it can affect men, too. A study of men confined to bed for 36 weeks found that they lost up to 39 percent of bone mass.

3 Do you play any sports?

Being active will certainly help keep you in good shape, and taking part in any sport is better than not doing so. For cardiovascular endurance (and general firming), both jogging and swimming rank very high, followed by cross-country skiing, bicycling, handball or squash, downhill skiing and basketball. But none of these sports, or any other, is really ideal for getting yourself into good shape overall. Jogging will give your legs a good workout; canoeing and kayaking will build your arms and shoulders. Swimming is the only sport that works nearly all the major muscle groups of the body. But no sport, not even swimming, will give all of your major muscles a thorough, balanced workout. In short, you cannot play yourself into good shape: You need shaping and toning exercises for that. And, if you do play sports, you will put heavy stresses on particular sets of muscles that should be strengthened before you engage in a sport.

4 Do you suffer from backache?

Nearly every adult American will suffer from backache at some point. But 80 percent of all backaches are preventable. Your back is affected by how you sit, stand, bend or twist. It can be thrown into spasm from stress, strain or sprain, from sleeping on the wrong mattress or from sitting in a badly adjusted seat. But weak, out-of-shape muscles are far more likely to be strained than strong, well-conditioned ones. For a program to avoid backache, see pages 79-93.

5 Are you doing exercises that might be harmful?

It is one thing to shape and tone your muscles — another thing to strain and tear them. Many people, with the best intentions in the world and with plenty of hard work, throw themselves into a conditioning program that damages their muscles. Before you undertake any exercises, check page 25 and make sure you do not do any of the harmful maneuvers shown there.

6 Do you keep breaking promises to yourself to get in shape?

As common sense might tell you, big, vague promises are hard to keep. Small, specific promises are easier to keep. Social psychologists call such small promises proximal goals. For instance, children may find it easier to learn a particular arithmetic lesson at hand than to worry about more distant goals. And adults might find it easier to settle on eight or 10 exercises to do every day than just to vow to "get in shape." And, if you miss your daily exercise, do not feel guilty. Just pick it up again the next day.

Use it or lose it

Exercise will keep you firm or get you firmer. But what if you do no exercise at all? What if, theoretically, your muscles did not even have to work against the force of gravity every day? In 1973, the nine Skylab astronauts lost between seven and 11 percent of their thigh-muscle volume while they were in space. One astronaut lost more than three pounds of leg muscle. Astronauts now do resistance-exercise routines in space, and they return with far less loss of muscle.

Sizing Yourself Up

Taking the Pinch Test

To be sure that your shaped and toned muscles will show, the first thing you need to do is discover whether excess fat is covering your muscles. The old-fashioned charts that show ideal weight as a function of height are of no use: They do not distinguish between muscle and fat. The easiest way to find out if you are carrying excess fat is to take the pinch test. Hold up one arm as though you were going to flex your biceps, but do not make a muscle. With the thumb and forefinger of your other hand, pinch the skin on the lower surface of your upper arm (just beneath the triceps). If the skin is more than 1/4- to 1/2-inch thick, you are a candidate for reducing your weight by cutting back on calories and stepping up your aerobic exercise.

Like a tailor-made suit, the exercises in this book can be fitted to your body. The better the fit, the more flattering the results will be.

How do you decide what exercises will do the most for your particular physique? First consider your body type. Long, thin ectomorphs must work a little harder to keep muscle. Mesomorphs, whose bodies tend toward the classic inverted V, develop more quickly. Plump endomorphs have naturally rounded contours.

Pure types do not exist, but they make it clear that our potentials do differ. A half-inch variation in the position where a tendon attaches to a bone can account for a 33 percent strength advantage, for example. The point is to compare yourself with yourself, not with other people, as you progress. Within the range of your potential, your results will depend on your motivation and performance, factors that you can control.

Now it is time to take the next step: an objective look at yourself standing nude before a full-length mirror. Without posing — pulling in your stomach or straightening up — consider your posture. Does your abdomen jut out? Does your lower back sway forward? Are your shoulders rounded? Is your upper chest sunken? Do you carry your head toward the front of your body?

Any "yes" answers are signs of bad posture. Though you may be able to hold yourself correctly for a minute or two, if you lack good muscle tone, you will inevitably sink back into the slump responsible for many lower back, neck and shoulder problems, as well as an unattractive appearance. But exercises for your abdominals, back and upper body, particularly the shoulder muscles, will tighten the loose connections that cause your sag. Rather than hanging limply, your skeleton will receive the muscular support it needs.

Now look for specific body areas with which you are dissatisfied. (Though spot reducing is impossible — and the places where you lose fat first are genetically programmed — you can firm specific areas, improving their appearance by toning underlying muscle.) In the following chapters, you will find exercises that can give you broader-looking shoulders; a firmer chest; tighter, more shapely inner and outer thighs; higher, firmer buttocks and flattering definition in your abdominals and elsewhere. The illustrations on pages 20 and 21 will help you choose the exercises you need.

Keep a notebook handy as you survey yourself. Record what you see, along with the date. This will be a motivational tool as well as a help in selecting exercises. You may use photos and a tape measure, too. Repeat this survey one month into your exercise program. By then, you will have begun to see results.

Test Your Strength

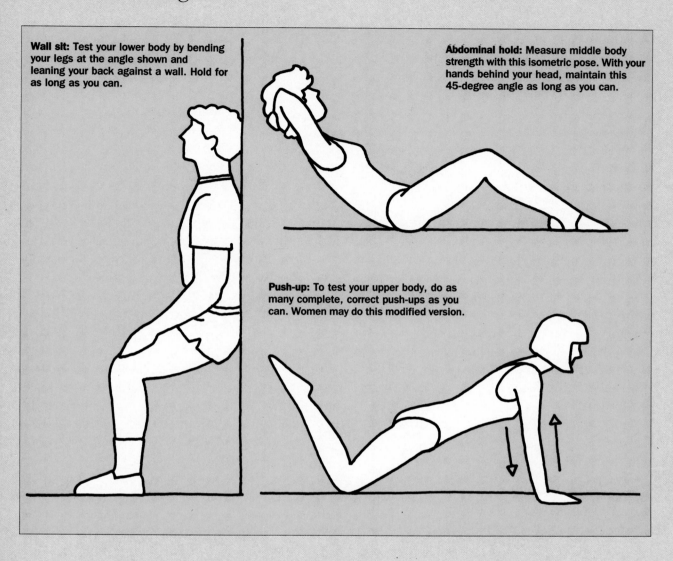

Wall sit: Test your lower body by bending your legs at the angle shown and leaning your back against a wall. Hold for as long as you can.

Abdominal hold: Measure middle body strength with this isometric pose. With your hands behind your head, maintain this 45-degree angle as long as you can.

Push-up: To test your upper body, do as many complete, correct push-ups as you can. Women may do this modified version.

One measure of muscle development is strength. The tests above assess the power in your lower, middle and upper body. Use the ratings below to gauge your own strength. If you are dissatisfied with your results, you can find help in the exercise chapters.

Wall sit
  Excellent - 90 seconds
  Good - 60 seconds
  Fair - 30 seconds
  Poor - less than 30 seconds

Abdominal hold
  Excellent - 25 seconds
  Good - 15 seconds
  Fair - 5 seconds
  Poor - less than 5 seconds

Push-ups
  Excellent - 25
  Good - 15
  Fair - 5
  Poor - fewer than 5

Choosing an Exercise

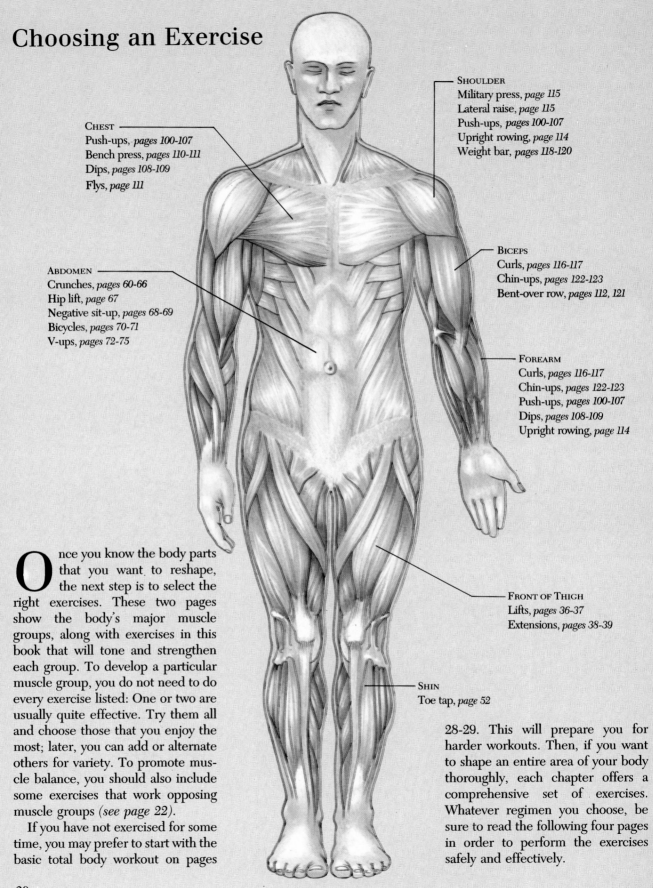

CHEST
Push-ups, *pages 100-107*
Bench press, *pages 110-111*
Dips, *pages 108-109*
Flys, *page 111*

SHOULDER
Military press, *page 115*
Lateral raise, *page 115*
Push-ups, *pages 100-107*
Upright rowing, *page 114*
Weight bar, *pages 118-120*

ABDOMEN
Crunches, *pages 60-66*
Hip lift, *page 67*
Negative sit-up, *pages 68-69*
Bicycles, *pages 70-71*
V-ups, *pages 72-75*

BICEPS
Curls, *pages 116-117*
Chin-ups, *pages 122-123*
Bent-over row, *pages 112, 121*

FOREARM
Curls, *pages 116-117*
Chin-ups, *pages 122-123*
Push-ups, *pages 100-107*
Dips, *pages 108-109*
Upright rowing, *page 114*

FRONT OF THIGH
Lifts, *pages 36-37*
Extensions, *pages 38-39*

SHIN
Toe tap, *page 52*

O nce you know the body parts that you want to reshape, the next step is to select the right exercises. These two pages show the body's major muscle groups, along with exercises in this book that will tone and strengthen each group. To develop a particular muscle group, you do not need to do every exercise listed: One or two are usually quite effective. Try them all and choose those that you enjoy the most; later, you can add or alternate others for variety. To promote muscle balance, you should also include some exercises that work opposing muscle groups *(see page 22)*.

If you have not exercised for some time, you may prefer to start with the basic total body workout on pages

28-29. This will prepare you for harder workouts. Then, if you want to shape an entire area of your body thoroughly, each chapter offers a comprehensive set of exercises. Whatever regimen you choose, be sure to read the following four pages in order to perform the exercises safely and effectively.

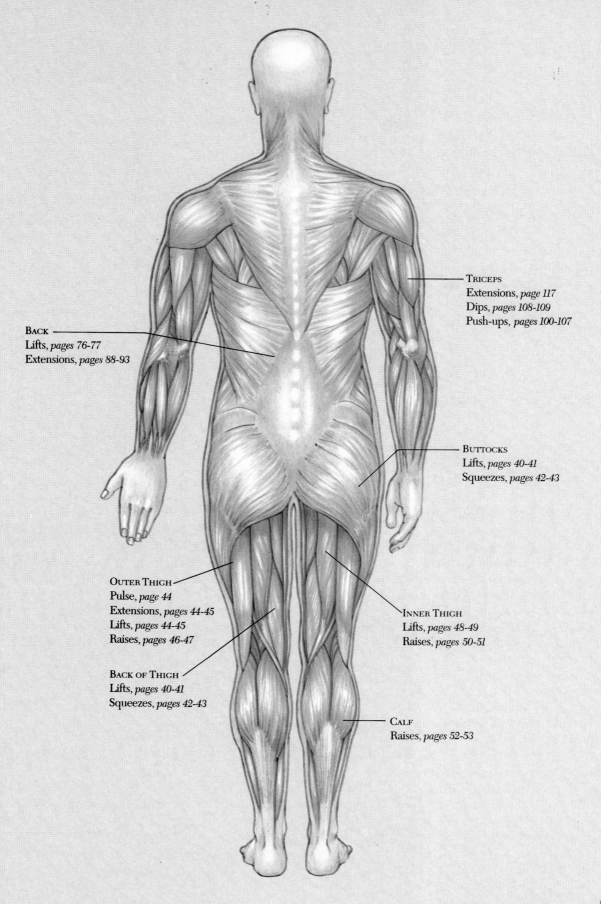

TRICEPS
Extensions, *page 117*
Dips, *pages 108-109*
Push-ups, *pages 100-107*

BACK
Lifts, *pages 76-77*
Extensions, *pages 88-93*

BUTTOCKS
Lifts, *pages 40-41*
Squeezes, *pages 42-43*

OUTER THIGH
Pulse, *page 44*
Extensions, *pages 44-45*
Lifts, *pages 44-45*
Raises, *pages 46-47*

INNER THIGH
Lifts, *pages 48-49*
Raises, *pages 50-51*

BACK OF THIGH
Lifts, *pages 40-41*
Squeezes, *pages 42-43*

CALF
Raises, *pages 52-53*

Training Keys You Need to Know

Overload. The only way to tone or strengthen a muscle is to place a greater-than-normal demand on it — that is, to overload it. As your muscles grow stronger, you must progressively increase the overload to continue improving. You can accomplish this by increasing how often, how long or how intensely you exercise.

Reps and sets. These are the building blocks of a workout. Reps are repetitions of an exercise: To do a push-up for eight reps means performing it eight times in a row before pausing or resting. A set is one string of reps followed by a rest interval. Performing eight push-ups, resting a minute, then doing eight more equals two sets.

Range of motion. A muscle's range of motion is the angle it covers when you extend or contract it. A good exercise allows you to move the muscle through its full range of motion, since partial movement can cause uneven development of the muscle or restrict the flexibility of your joints.

Muscle balance. To work only some muscle groups and ignore others invites injury and a lack of proportion in the area of the muscle. The key is to work muscles on opposite sides of a joint. Examples of opposing muscles are biceps and triceps in the upper arm; quadriceps and hamstrings in the thigh; and pectorals and latissimus dorsi in the torso.

The Training Regimen

HOW OFTEN

Studies show that you should exercise a muscle three to four times each week to achieve solid muscle tone. Exercising more than that may speed up your progress somewhat. But be careful not to wear yourself out. Experienced body builders who work out five or six days a week exercise different muscle groups on successive days, typically alternating between lower body and upper body.

HOW LONG

The length of a training session will vary, depending upon what you want to accomplish. A starting workout of eight or 10 basic exercises, such as the ones on pages 28-29, can take 20 to 30 minutes. A more advanced program will include additional exercises for one or more body parts (though you can skip working those muscles that are already firm from other forms of exercise). If your workouts exceed 45 minutes, consider splitting them up and exercising more frequently. For example, you might train five times a week: three sessions devoted to upper body work, alternating with two sessions of exercises for the trunk and legs. This will prevent you from becoming exhausted and will add variety to your regimen. You can also vary the pace of workouts, pushing hard and fast on some days, slower and easier on others.

HOW HARD

Do three sets of 10 repetitions each: That is the way to build shape and tone in a muscle.

Take it easy at first. If you have not exercised for some time, start with a few reps of the easiest versions of each exercise. Gradually work up to 10 reps without straining.

Once you can do 10, rest a minute, then start a second set. After a few weeks, you should do 10 reps on the second set and be able to start on the third. This last set should thoroughly tire the muscles.

As your strength improves so that doing three sets no longer brings you to the point of fatigue, you can continue to overload the muscles in several ways:

1. Make the exercise harder. Many of the basic exercises in this book include variations that increase the load of your body weight on working muscles. With exercises involving weights, you can increase the amount of weight.

2. Decrease the rest interval between sets. With less time to rest, muscles must work harder to lift the same amount of weight.

3. Increase the number of repetitions in the last set. This will continue to improve your muscle tone. And as you exceed 10 repetitions, an increase in absolute strength or muscle size gives way to gains in muscular endurance, which enables your muscles to make a sustained effort.

Ten Guidelines for Working Out

1. WARM UP.

A five- to 10-minute warm-up increases blood flow and helps prevent soreness and strains in muscles, tendons and ligaments. In each of the following three chapters, the exercise section is preceded by a stretching-and-limbering routine.

2. WORK LARGER MUSCLES FIRST.

The big muscles of the legs, chest and back often require heavier workloads in an exercise to achieve any result. So it is best to exercise them before cumulative fatigue starts to build. Exercising these muscles first also helps your body to continue to warm up.

3. PAIR YOUR EXERCISES.

Arrange your routine so that you work one muscle group, then its opposite. For example, pair quadriceps lifts with extensions for the hamstrings, biceps curls with dips for the triceps, and push-ups for the chest and shoulders with bent-over rows or chin-ups that work the latissimus. By performing exercises in pairs, you also allow each muscle group to recover in case you want to work it in a second exercise.

4. USE VARIATIONS CAREFULLY.

In many instances, you can perform slight variations on the basic movement of an exercise. These not only afford variety, but can increase the intensity or focus of an exercise. However, during any one workout, it is better to do distinctly different exercises than several variations of one exercise. Performing three versions of a push-up, for example, is not as effective as doing one type of push-up and, later, a bench press or overhead row. By all means, take advantage of variations, but from one workout to the next.

5. WORK SLOWLY AND STEADILY.

Slow, controlled movement subjects the muscle to relatively consistent stress during both the lifting and the lowering phase of an exercise. Quick, explosive movements make you work hard at the beginning of a repetition. But that initial thrust can then carry the muscle through the rest of its motion. As well as being less productive for shaping and toning, fast movements are also more likely to injure you.

6. BREATHE EVENLY.

You may need to hold your breath briefly during an instant of effort. But do not hold it longer than a second or two: Though your muscles may be working anaerobically, holding your breath too long can prevent blood from returning to the heart. Holding your breath can also cause cramping during abdominal work.

7. USE A FULL RANGE OF MOTION.

For each rep, move the joint through its maximum extension and flexion. A muscle that makes only a partial movement performs less work and can lose flexibility. Because range of motion can differ for each joint and each exercise, you need to concentrate in each case on what your own maximum is. Do not flex or extend so far that the joint is suddenly bearing the workload: That should always be the job of the muscle.

8. REST BETWEEN SETS.

After the first set, you need to restore energy to the muscle so that it can continue to contract during the next set. If the rest interval is too short, you will exhaust yourself; if too long, the next set will not make you work harder (which it should). For most training purposes, one to two minutes are sufficient. But if you are performing only one set of an exercise, you need to rest only a few seconds before starting an exercise that stresses a different muscle group.

9. COOL DOWN.

Abruptly stopping a workout can cause blood to pool in the veins, creating a sudden drop in blood pressure that may produce light-headedness or fainting. An activity such as running in place or repeating one of the warm-up routines keeps blood circulating and helps the muscles recover.

10. KEEP TRACK OF YOUR PROGRESS.

Record reps, sets and weights for each exercise every week. Some muscles will respond more quickly than others, so you will need to increase the overload for exercises at different rates. Every month, retest your strength *(page 18)* and reassess your appearance. Once you have achieved the look and the strength you want, you need not increase the workload further. But you do have to keep working out to maintain the benefits.

Common Mistakes

The human body differs from other machines in that it improves with use. But exercise can break down your body rather than tone it if you are not careful. The three most common errors are to do bad exercises that may actually be harmful, to do good exercises incorrectly and to overdo good exercises.

The exercises on the opposite page are bad ones that people do routinely. Most of them do not provide the benefits they are intended to, and each is quite capable of causing injury to muscles, tendons and ligaments. Some of them have been standard exercises in schools for years, and some are still used in fitness classes. In each case, this book presents a better, safer alternative.

Choosing the right exercises but performing them incorrectly can be just as bad. If you do not maintain the correct position all through an exercise, you may fail to work the muscles you intended to. Worse, you may injure yourself by placing strain where it does not belong.

Another common mistake is to overtax your muscles, especially at the beginning of a program. Pushing muscles to their limits before they have become accustomed to exercise is almost certain to result in soreness. For an exercise to work, it should require some effort, but not strain or pain. Do not persist with any exercise that hurts, especially if the discomfort you feel is in the joints. You should feel the effort in your muscles, not your joints.

Muscles can be damaged by incautious exercise. Extreme overexertion, particularly when muscles have not been properly warmed up, may literally tear muscle fibers.

Minor muscle soreness can often be relieved by a hot bath or a massage. Muscle or joint strain may be treated with ice bags. But persistent joint pain calls for a doctor's care.

If muscles are severely or persistently sore, the cause is probably overtraining. Other signs of serious overexertion include excessive fatigue, listlessness, depression and difficulty in sleeping. If you have these symptoms and have been exercising, you may need more rest each day.

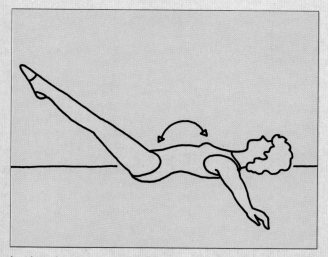

Leg lowering arches the lower back, placing it under dangerous stress. Instead, do the bicycle *(pages 70-71)*.

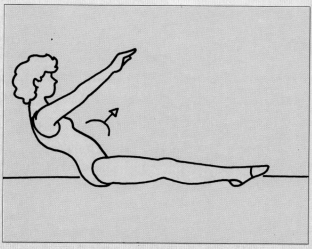

Straight-leg sit-ups also force your back to arch, overstressing it. Try the crunch *(pages 60-66)*.

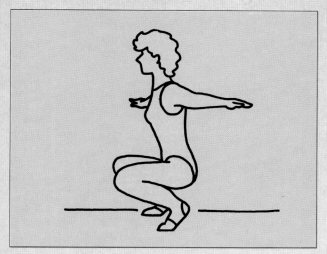

The duck walk strains your knees. It may even rupture your ligaments. Choose quadriceps lifts *(pages 36-37)*.

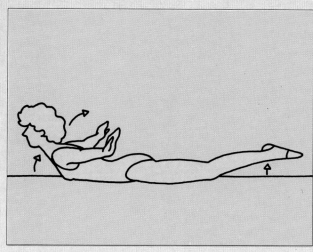

Back arching dangerously shortens muscles that usually need lengthening. Use a safe back exercise *(pages 92-93)*.

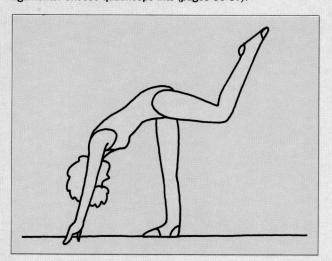

Locking your supporting knee in the donkey kick imperils your sacroiliac. Do hamstring and gluteal lifts instead *(pages 40-41)*.

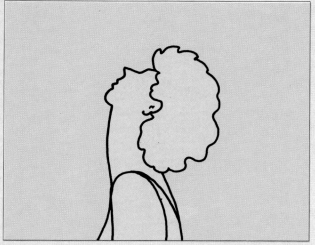

Bending your head back hard in the neck roll may hurt your spine. The seated back lift *(page 76)* builds neck strength safely.

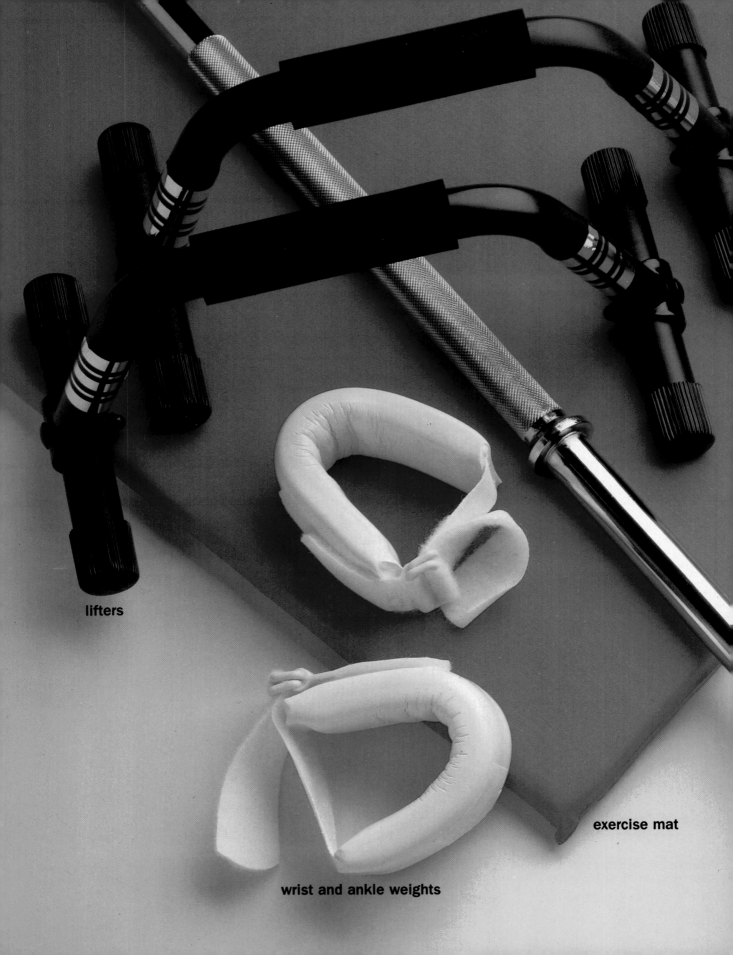

lifters

wrist and ankle weights

exercise mat

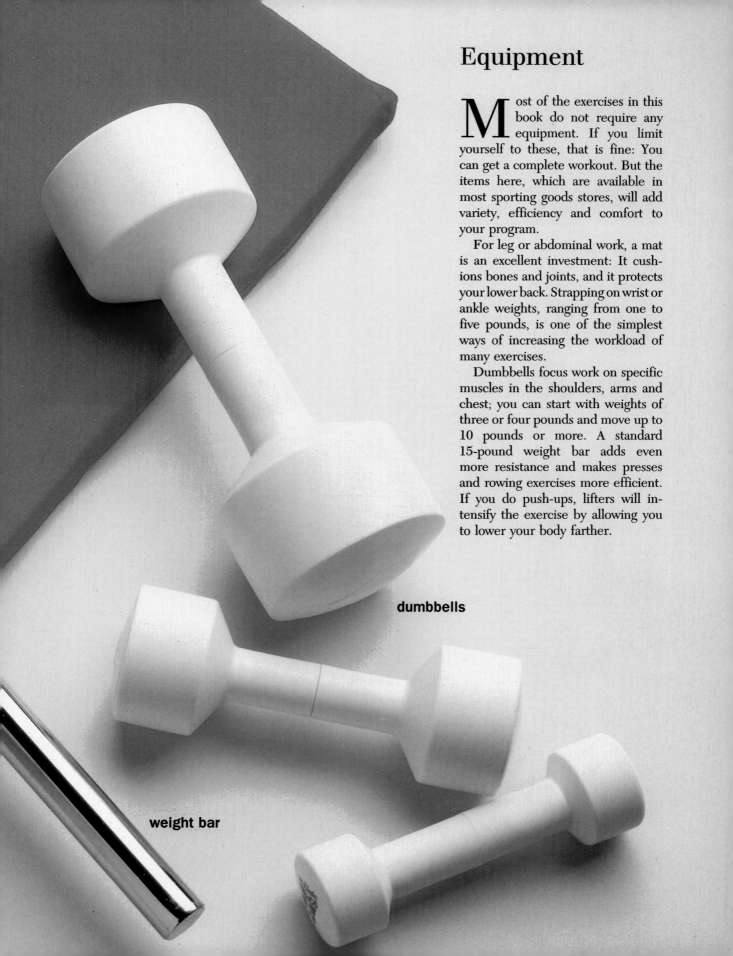

Equipment

Most of the exercises in this book do not require any equipment. If you limit yourself to these, that is fine: You can get a complete workout. But the items here, which are available in most sporting goods stores, will add variety, efficiency and comfort to your program.

For leg or abdominal work, a mat is an excellent investment: It cushions bones and joints, and it protects your lower back. Strapping on wrist or ankle weights, ranging from one to five pounds, is one of the simplest ways of increasing the workload of many exercises.

Dumbbells focus work on specific muscles in the shoulders, arms and chest; you can start with weights of three or four pounds and move up to 10 pounds or more. A standard 15-pound weight bar adds even more resistance and makes presses and rowing exercises more efficient. If you do push-ups, lifters will intensify the exercise by allowing you to lower your body farther.

dumbbells

weight bar

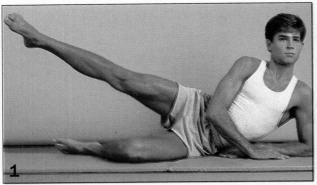

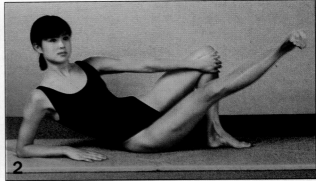

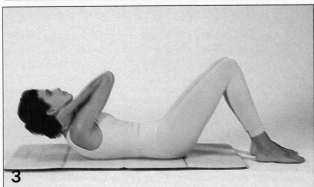

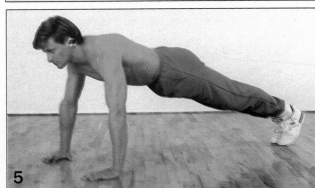

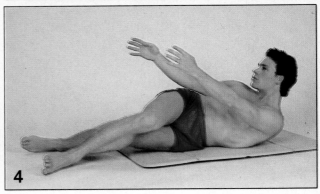

1. Outer-thigh raise, *page 46*
2. Inner-thigh raise, *pages 50-51*
3. Crunch, *pages 60-61*
4. Diagonal crunch, *page 63*
5. Push-up, *pages 102-103*
6. Upright rowing, *pages 114, 119*
7. Bent-over rowing, *pages 112, 121*
8. Dip, *page 108*

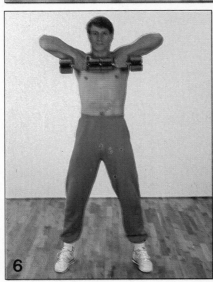

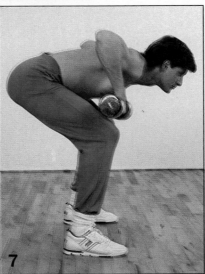

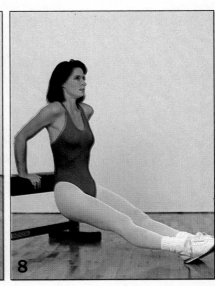

A Basic Workout

I f you are out of shape and pressed for time, doing the eight exercises shown opposite will start getting you into good overall shape. To isolate certain muscles or for more advanced workouts, you need to turn to the following three chapters. But this workout brings all of the major muscle groups into play, and it takes only 30 minutes. Performing it three times a week should quickly improve your general appearance and strength.

The routine is designed to follow the principles of resistance training. It works from large muscles to small and provides work for both sides of opposing muscle groups. If you have a special interest in shaping your thighs, you may start your routine with the two exercises to the right. If you want extra work for your upper arms, do the curl and lift below after completing the first eight.

To learn more about the exercises and how to perform them correctly, turn to the pages indicated. Be sure to warm up before your workout.

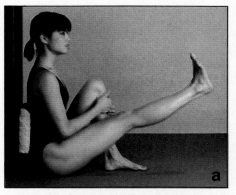

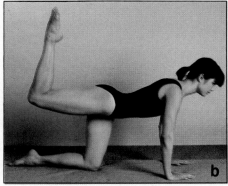

A. Quadriceps lift, *pages 36-37*
B. Hamstring and gluteal lift, *pages 40-41*

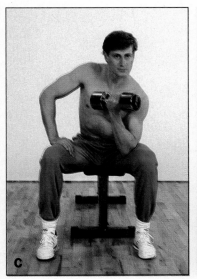

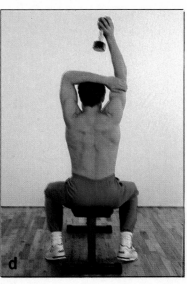

C. Concentration curl, *pages 116-117*
D. Triceps extension, *page 117*

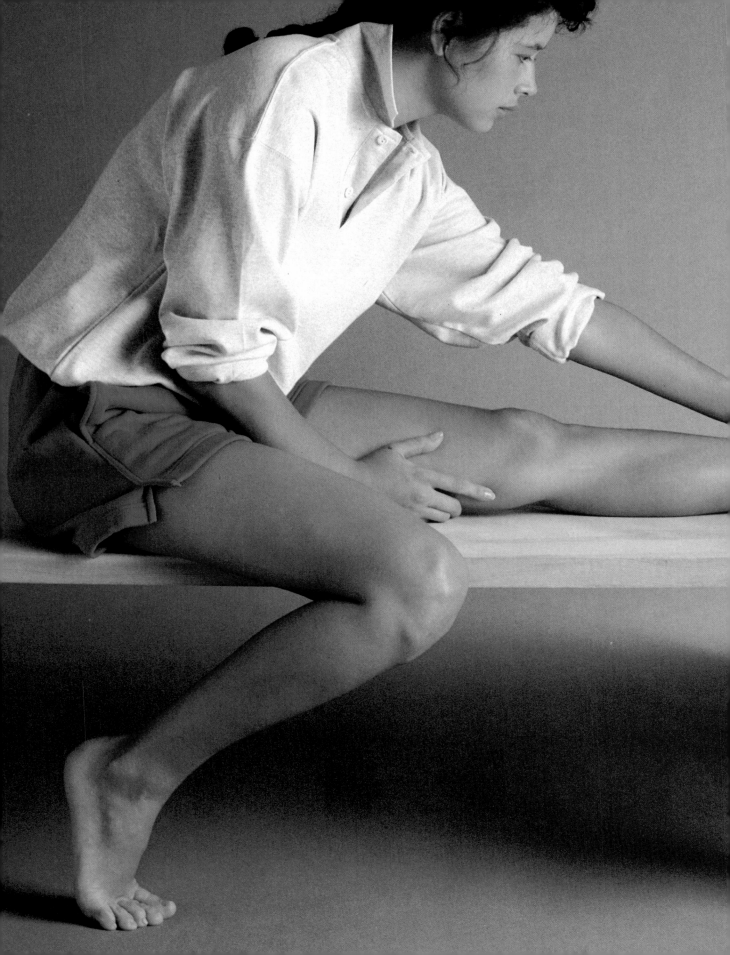

CHAPTER TWO

The Lower Body

*Powerful exercises for your body's
biggest muscles*

Your largest muscles — and potentially the best-developed ones — are likely to be in your lower body. The reason is simple: Your legs and hips have to support and move the rest of your body. For most adults, that means carrying more than 100 pounds.

Powerful musculature does not guarantee, however, that the lower body can be shaped or toned more readily than other parts of the body. In fact, your lower body can be slower to show the effects of exercise. Precisely because of their power, the body's large, high-use muscles may barely be stressed during an exercise that would easily overload smaller, less active muscles. If, on the other hand, lower body muscles have become slack from underuse, their size makes the resulting sag more noticeable.

Thighs and hips tend to be sites not only for oversized muscles, but also for accumulated fat. This is often a concern for women, whose hormones cause fat to collect in this area. (Male hormones predispose

31

men to store fat around the waist.) Many women feel especially self-conscious about the condition called cellulite, the dimply ripples that appear on thighs and buttocks. Some women are convinced that removing it calls for special lotions and creams. Lotions do not affect cellulite, however, nor does any other treatment, because cellulite is nothing but ordinary fat. This fat may seem to be more stubborn than fat in the upper body, but that is only because there is more of it; the upper body usually has a thinner fat layer between muscle and skin.

Muscle-toning exercises alone will not slim your thighs, but such exercises can improve your appearance by firming and shaping underlying muscle tissue as you shed weight. The only way to lose fat and get rid of unsightly bulges is to decrease your caloric intake through dieting and increase your caloric or energy output through such aerobic exercises as brisk walking, running, swimming or cycling. However, while aerobic exercise tones some muscles in your lower body, it may leave other major lower body muscles virtually unused.

Research has shown that the gluteus maximus, the muscle that underlies and shapes the buttocks, works very little during walking, even brisk aerobic walking. Running, cycling and lifting a heavy weight from a squatting position do not significantly activate this muscle, either. Nor do any of these activities have much impact on the muscles of the inner thigh. Instead, you need to perform such exercises as those on pages 40-43 and 48-49, which work just these areas.

A look at the anatomy of the lower body *(see illustration opposite)* indicates how exercises targeted at specific muscles can effectively firm thighs and hips. The body's center of gravity is located in the pelvis, and muscles on the outside of the hips balance and support the torso and move the legs. These muscles are most efficiently toned by leg exercises. Inside the pelvis, powerful hip flexors, the strongest muscles in the body, steady hips and thighs as well as move them. Generally, these muscles do not need strengthening: Most people benefit more from developing the abdominals that oppose them.

The quadriceps, a four-part muscle, is the principal shaper of your thigh and supplies much of the power in forward movement. It is used whenever you jump, run, kick, skip, lift or push. Besides improving sports performance, training your quads makes it easier to lift objects from the floor the safe way — with your legs, rather than your back, providing most of the power.

The quadriceps is also important to the knee, a joint particularly vulnerable to injury because it allows movement only in a semicircular plane. This limited rotation gives great stability to the lower body, but it exposes the joint to danger whenever force comes from another direction. By strengthening the quadriceps, the main connection in this hinge, you can reinforce, protect and strengthen your knees.

On the back of your thigh, the hamstrings, a three-part muscle, opposes the quad with help from the gluteals. Hamstring pulls and tears are among the most common and serious sports injuries. Exercises such as sprinting and jumping build such mighty quads that they

Lower Body

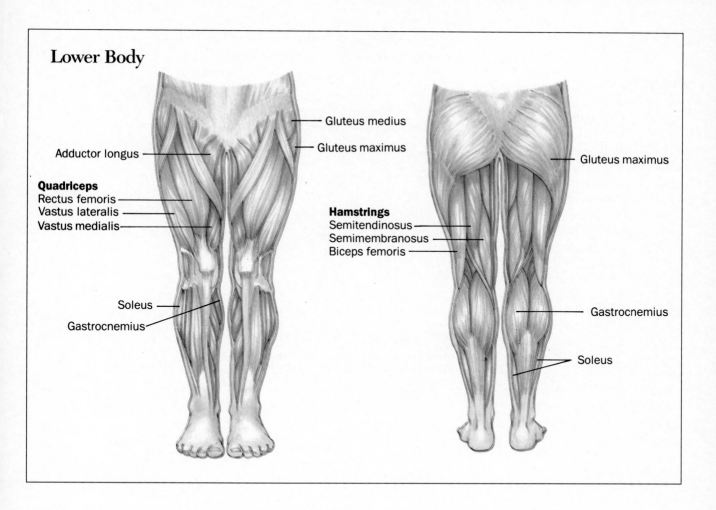

Adductor longus

Gluteus medius

Gluteus maximus

Gluteus maximus

Quadriceps
Rectus femoris
Vastus lateralis
Vastus medialis

Hamstrings
Semitendinosus
Semimembranosus
Biceps femoris

Soleus

Gastrocnemius

Gastrocnemius

Soleus

can literally tear weak hamstrings apart if these opposing muscles fail to relax when the quads contract. Normally hamstrings need only be two thirds as strong as the quadriceps. But they must be at least that strong, and in many people, they are not.

The muscles that line the side of hip and thigh lift your leg away from your body and rotate it inward. These are the abductors. One major abductor is the gluteus medius. If this muscle is toned, you can feel it under your hands when they are placed on your hips with your fingers touching the bumps on the front of your hip bones.

The big muscles of your calf, the gastrocnemius and the soleus, join at the Achilles tendon fixed to your heel. These muscles pull on your heel, allowing you to rise on your toes as you walk or run. On the front of the shin are muscles that lift feet and toes. Exercises for the muscles of the lower leg help protect the shin and the ankle, frequent sites of injuries from physical activity.

In the section that follows, you can choose exercises to tone one particular area, though they should be balanced with work for the opposing muscle group. For example, toe taps for the shin should accompany calf raises. Or you can choose one or two exercises for each muscle group to firm and strengthen all of your lower body.

Warm-Ups

The warm-ups and stretches here prepare your entire lower body, including commonly neglected areas such as inner thighs, for the exercises that follow.

Be sure to stretch your lower body muscles before you begin toning. This prevents shortening, which makes muscles more likely to tear and is particularly dangerous in lower body muscles, since these receive a great deal of stress in daily life. .

The stretches here loosen muscles and joints that grow stiff without such special attention. They target hip joints, the lower back and thigh muscles, all of which tend to get tight when the lower body is strengthened. The final four exercises, starting with the on-the-back hamstring stretch, should be repeated as a cool-down when you have finished your lower body workout. They will keep your muscles from losing elasticity.

You should never stretch or work muscles that are cold. First, run in place for several minutes to accelerate your heart rate and start blood flowing faster to the muscles you intend to strengthen. Then perform the routine on these two pages.

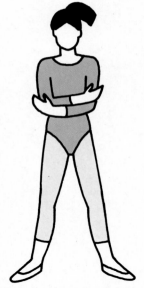
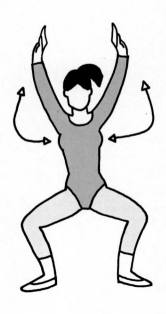

Fold your arms *(above)*, bend your knees, gently swing your arms down, then overhead in a U *(right)*. Reverse the swing with legs straight. Repeat 20 times.

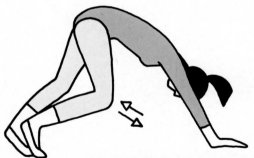

Rhythmically bend one knee, then the other. Keep your buttocks high, your knees unlocked. Flex each leg 10 times.

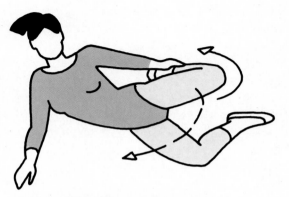

Hold your ankle and pull your upper leg back to stretch your quadriceps. Hold for 20 seconds. Swing your leg to the front to loosen your hip. Repeat on other side.

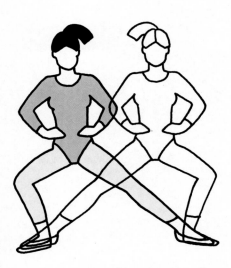

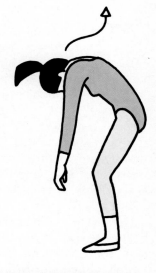

Take a wide stance with your feet turned out. With hands on hips, slowly lunge first right, then left, 10 times to each side.

Bend forward, letting your entire upper body hang loosely, including your head. With knees bent, curl up slowly.

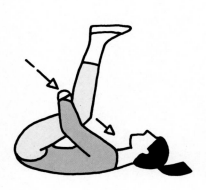

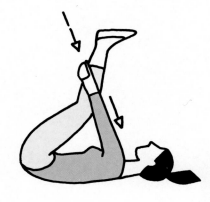

To stretch hamstrings, lie on your back with your hands clasped around the backs of your knees. Pull gently toward your torso for about 20 seconds. Clasp hands behind your calves and pull for 20 seconds more.

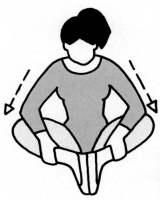

Press your left elbow against the outside of your right knee. Turn your head and torso as far as you are able. Hold for 20 seconds. Repeat on other side.

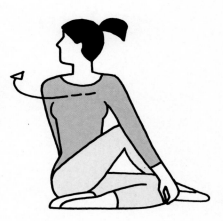

Put the soles of your feet together and your hands on your lower legs. Lean forward from the hips and let your weight loosen your thigh muscles. Hold for 20 seconds.

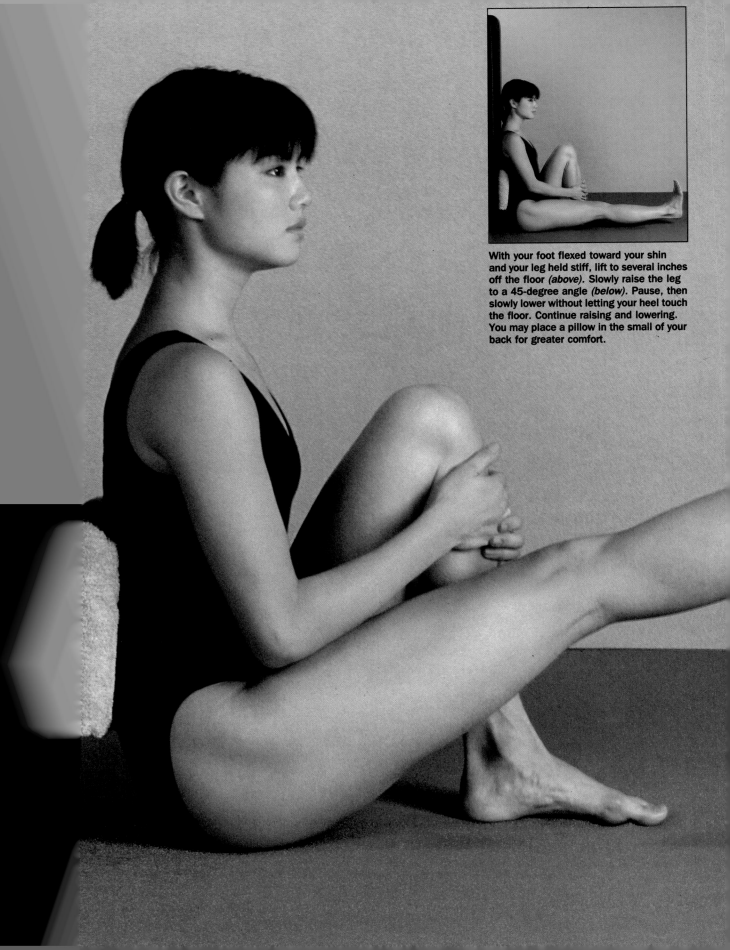

With your foot flexed toward your shin and your leg held stiff, lift to several inches off the floor *(above)*. Slowly raise the leg to a 45-degree angle *(below)*. Pause, then slowly lower without letting your heel touch the floor. Continue raising and lowering. You may place a pillow in the small of your back for greater comfort.

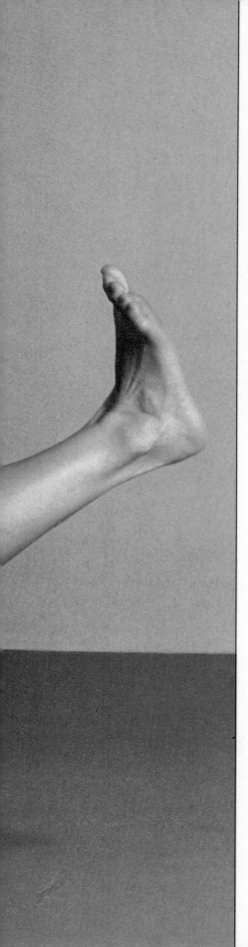

Quadriceps Lifts

Toning the quadriceps, the major muscle underpinning the front and sides of your thigh, shapes your upper leg more effectively than any other exercise. A muscle that performs two jobs — straightening the leg and raising it — the quadriceps can be trained either by flexing the thigh on the hip or by extending the leg below the knee. Straight-leg quad lifts, like the ones shown here, strengthen the front of the quad, the rectus femoris, both ways. (Keeping your knee stiff makes the quad perform its straightening function.)

Do one lift and one extension. If you are a beginner, do the exercises lying on your back. Work up to the seated versions, which shape and strengthen faster. Beginners should alternate legs between sets. If you are at a more advanced level, do all three sets for each leg before switching. As you progress, add one- or two-pound ankle weights. If you want even more development, add up to five-pound weights to all quad exercises. If you cannot keep your knee straight in the lifts or extend it fully in the extensions, reduce the weights. (People with back pain, however, should not add weights.)

Straight-leg quad lifts are a good choice if your knees are vulnerable to injury or have been injured. Start strengthening with the lifts shown here (with your doctor's approval). When you no longer feel pain or instability in the injured joint, add one of the lower-leg extensions shown on the next two pages.

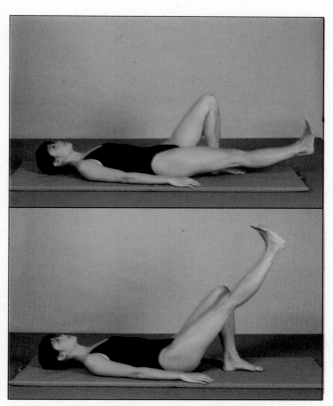

Flatten your lower back against the floor *(top)*, then slowly raise and lower your leg vertically. Do not let your leg rest on the floor. Keep your knee extended, your ankle flexed and your toes up.

Quadriceps Extensions

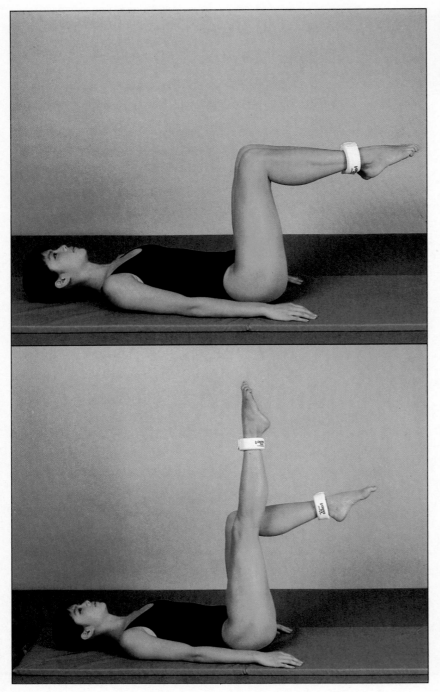

Lie with your lower back flat on the floor, your thighs and calves at right angles and your toes pointed *(top left)*. Straighten one leg so that your toe points toward the ceiling *(bottom left)*; slowly lower to the first position. Your hips should not move.

Sit on the edge of a bench or chair with your back straight *(inset right)*. Lift one leg off the floor *(opposite)*, then fully extend it. Return to the first position, keeping your foot flexed. Avoid tilting or moving your pelvis, or tensing your upper body.

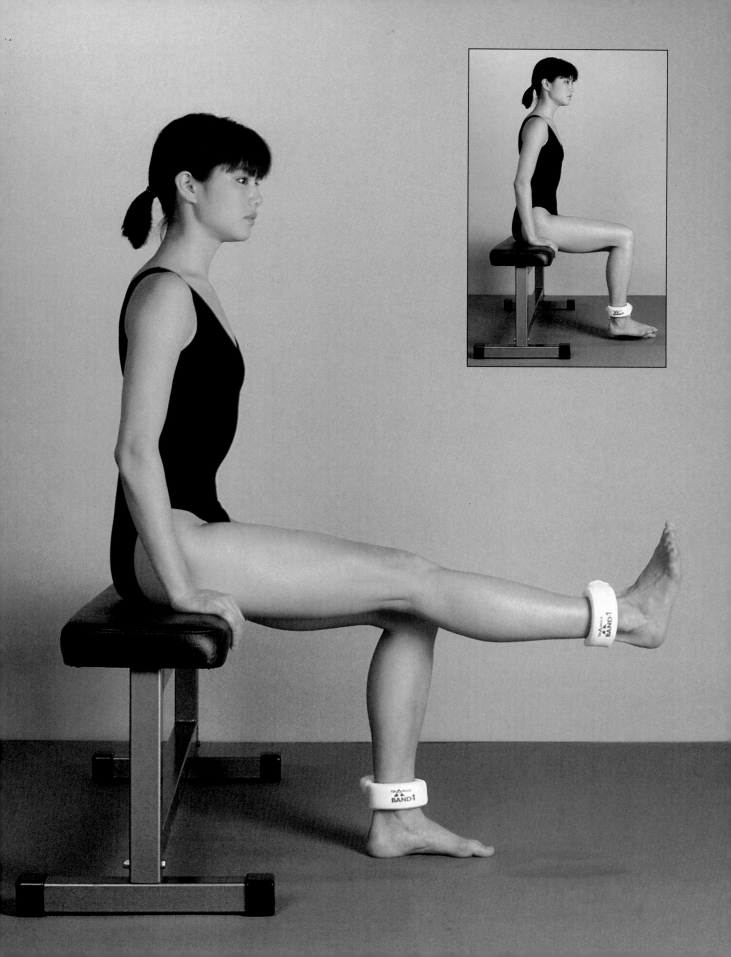

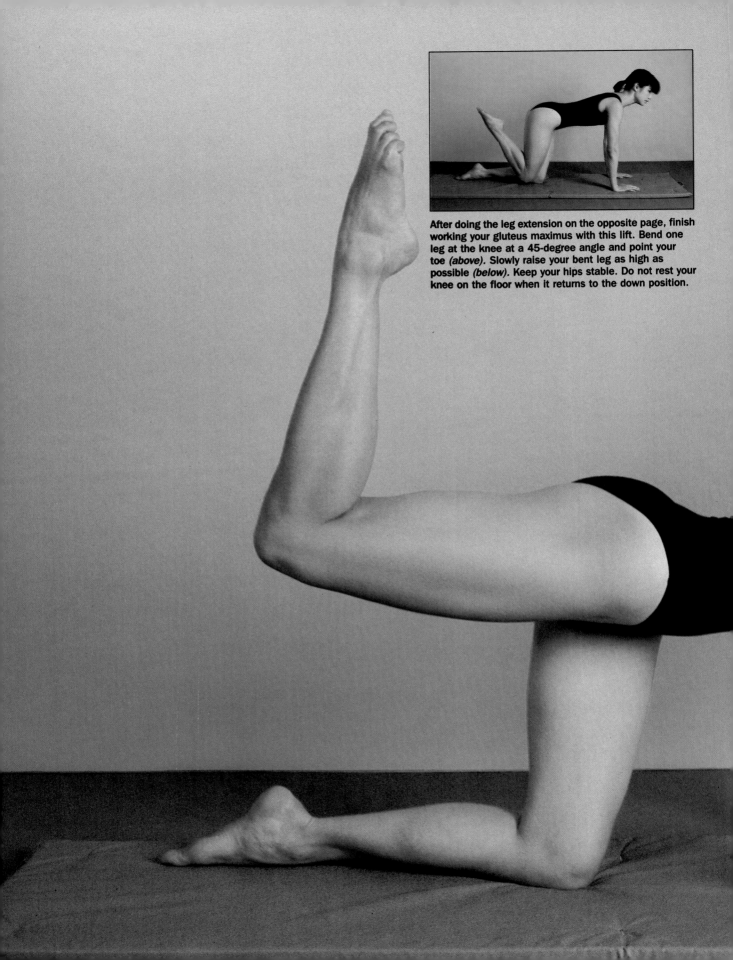

After doing the leg extension on the opposite page, finish working your gluteus maximus with this lift. Bend one leg at the knee at a 45-degree angle and point your toe *(above)*. Slowly raise your bent leg as high as possible *(below)*. Keep your hips stable. Do not rest your knee on the floor when it returns to the down position.

Hamstring and Gluteal Lifts

Working your hamstrings and gluteals will balance quad work, protect vulnerable hamstrings and continue the toning you began in the front of your thigh.

First do the leg extensions below, then finish with the bent-leg lifts at left. As with the quadriceps exercises, beginners should switch legs after each set; those who are more advanced should do two to three sets in a row for each leg. Add ankle weights as you grow stronger. The buttocks and hamstrings exercises on the following two pages work the same muscles. Choose them for variety or if you have back problems. (Their reclining position supports the back.)

Place your hands directly below your shoulders. Extend one leg straight back with your toes pointed (below); bring your lower leg up to a right angle as you flex your foot (bottom). Keep your torso steady.

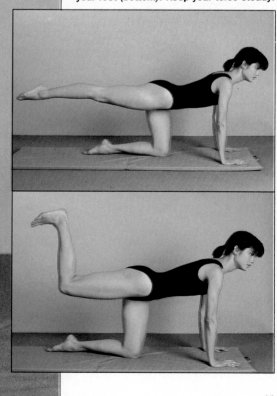

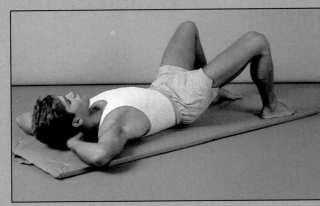

Get into position with your back flat on the floor, your upper body relaxed, your feet separated and your knees bent. Tilt your pelvis, raising your hips slightly *(above)*. Do not raise your upper back off the floor. Press your legs together tightly, squeezing your buttocks hard *(below)*. Hold. Separate your knees and repeat.

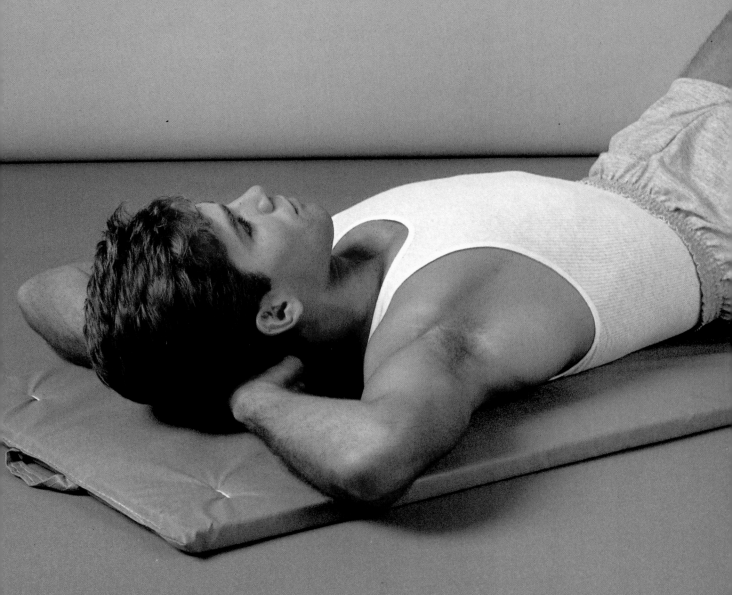

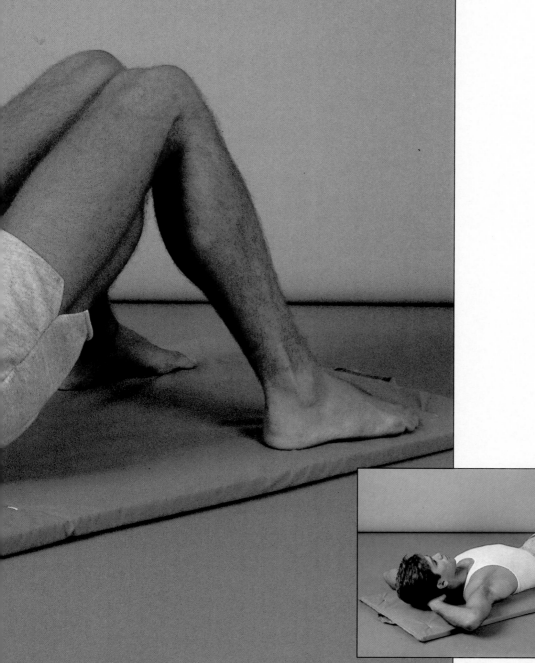

Hamstring and Gluteal Squeezes

With your feet and knees together, lift your hips, leaving your upper back on the floor *(above)*. Squeeze thighs and buttocks tightly. Hold, lower slowly and relax.

43

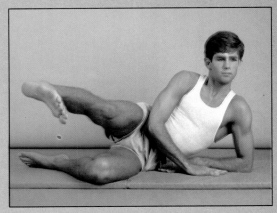

With your supporting leg bent at a right angle to your body, hold your upper leg straight out parallel to your thigh *(above)*. Keep your lifted foot flexed. Make sure that your leg is rotated so that your heel is up and your toe down. Pulse your heel out slowly and rhythmically. (At about the rate of your heartbeat, tighten your leg muscles and press your heel out hard, then relax the muscles.) For extensions, keep the same position and bend your upper knee, drawing your lower leg in until it is directly above your bottom leg *(below)*. Then extend it fully to the starting position.

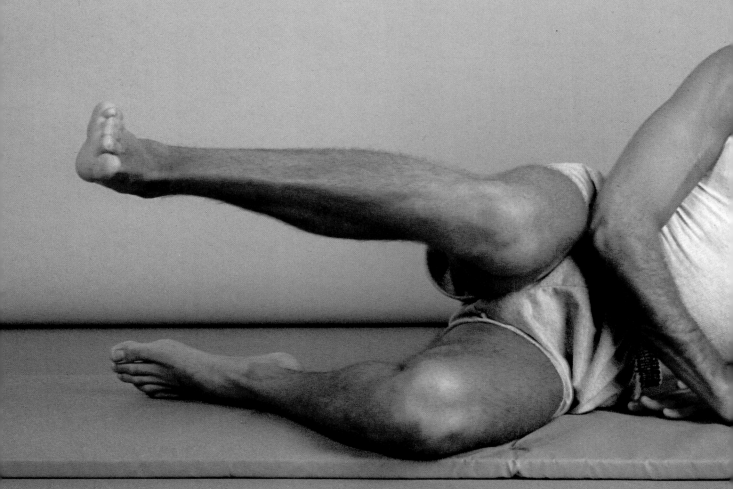

Outer-Thigh Work

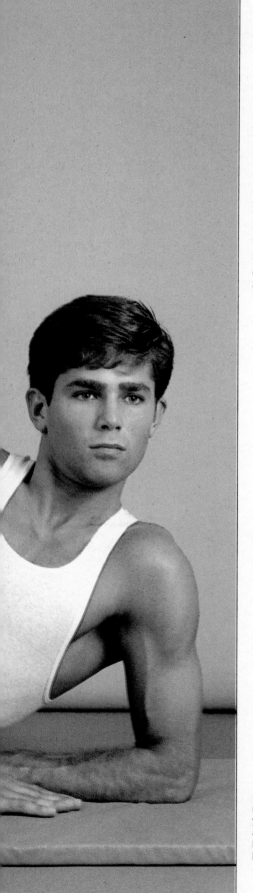

Lifting your leg to the side firms not only your outer thigh, but also the side of your hip. That is the site of the gluteus medius, your second largest gluteal muscle and one of your major thigh abductors. The exercises on these two pages give you a comprehensive outer-thigh- and outer-hip-firming routine. Work them as a three-exercise set. The pulses *(inset)*, alternately tensing and relaxing, concentrate effort in the gluteals; then the extensions *(below, oppo-* *site)* work all the abductors. Finally, the bent-leg lifts *(below)* isolate the outer thigh.

The straight-leg raises on the following two pages are also a classic way to work the outer thigh and gluteus medius. You may do them as an alternative. In all outer-thigh work, position is crucial. If you do these exercises wrong, you will end up working the quadriceps, rather than the abductors, or straining your lower back. As you progress, add ankle weights for extra resistance.

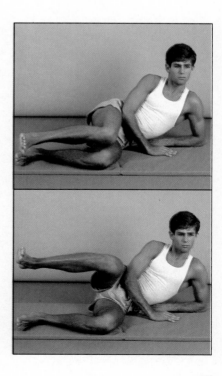

Finish with bent-leg lifts. Let your legs remain at right angles to your body with your ankles flexed *(top right)*. Slowly raise and lower your upper leg *(bottom right)*. Do not let it rest in the down position between lifts.

Outer-Thigh Raises

Resting on your forearm and hip, with your bottom leg bent at a 90-degree angle and your top leg raised slightly *(inset)*, slowly lift and lower your top leg in a straight line with your body. Keep your upper body erect and your foot flexed.

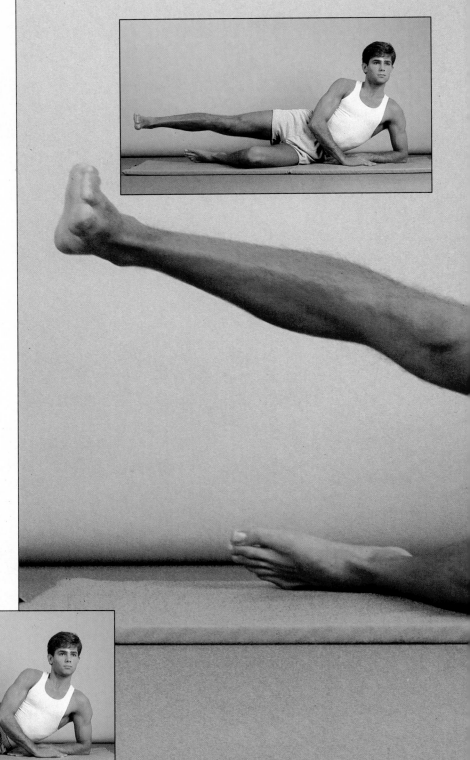

Starting in the position shown in inset photo, repeat the lifting and lowering, but with your toe pointed *(above)*. Do not allow your body to slump or your leg to rotate upward.

46

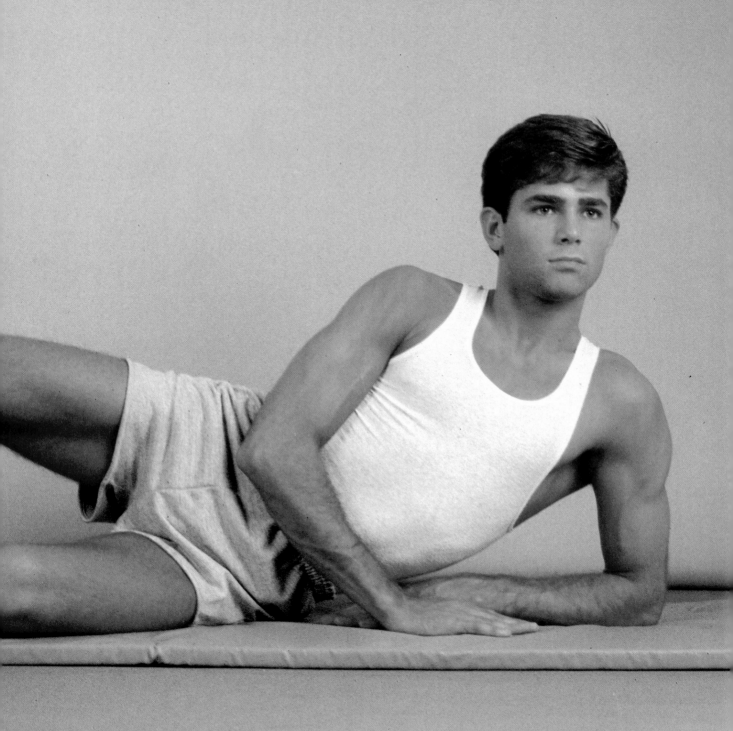

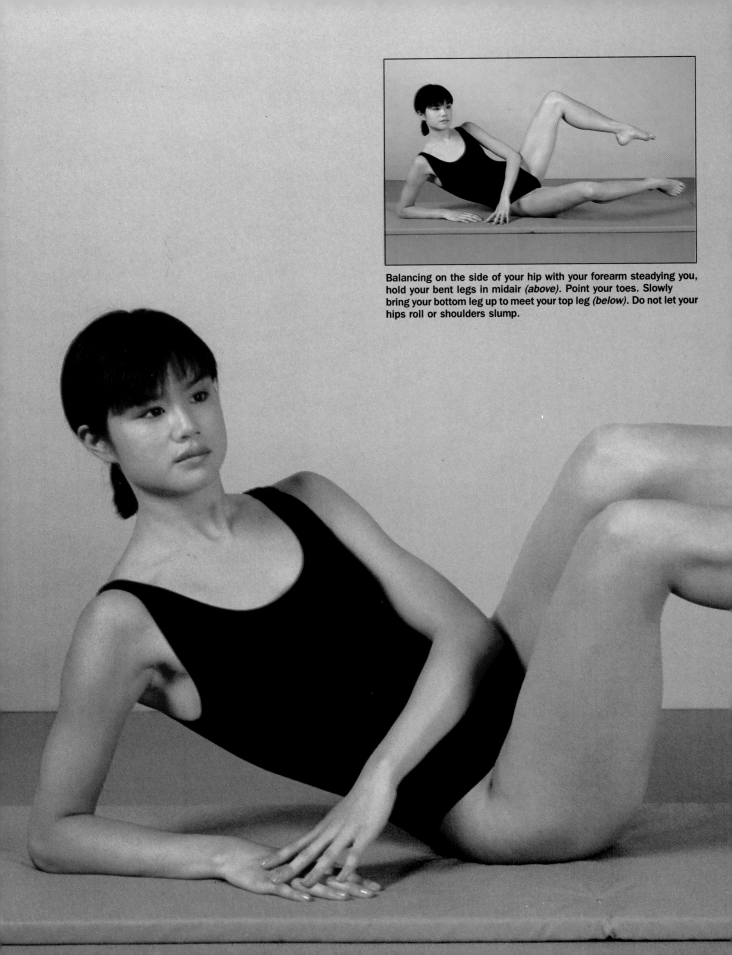

Balancing on the side of your hip with your forearm steadying you, hold your bent legs in midair *(above)*. Point your toes. Slowly bring your bottom leg up to meet your top leg *(below)*. Do not let your hips roll or shoulders slump.

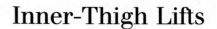

Inner-Thigh Lifts

Because they are an under-exercised area, the inner thighs show one of the quickest responses to toning exercises of any lower body area. To begin firming your inner thighs, do the leg-fanning exercise below. It is the easiest and the safest, particularly for anyone troubled by back pain or weak knees. The hip lift at left should be added as soon as you are able: It stresses the muscles in a slightly different way. After you have built up some strength, you can do the inner-thigh leg raises on the following two pages. If you have adequate flexibility, do the raises with your leg behind the bent leg.

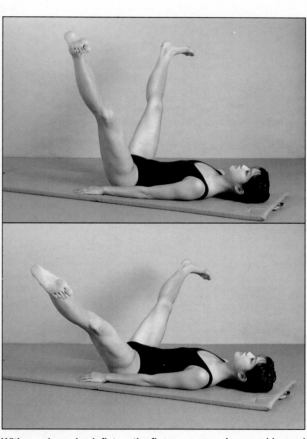

With your lower back flat on the floor, your arms by your sides and your upper body relaxed, lift your legs to form a V over your hips *(top)*. Separate them as widely as you can without pain *(above)*, then draw them back into the starting V.

Inner-Thigh Raises

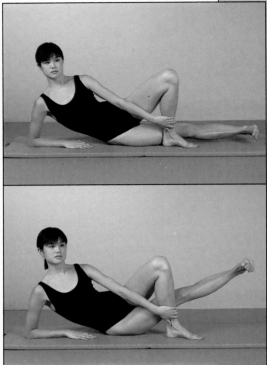

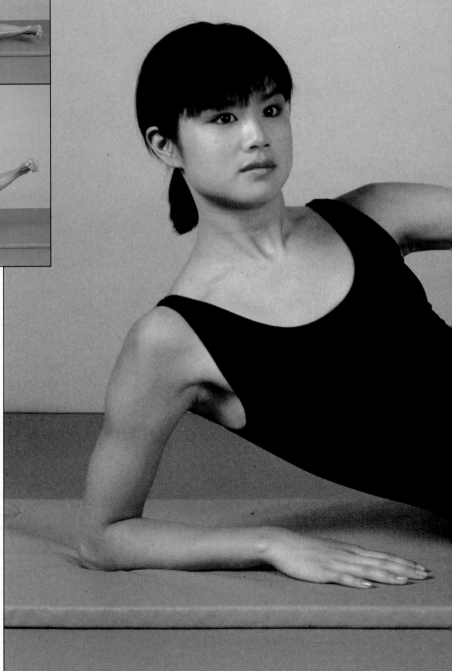

The most difficult inner-thigh raise
and the fastest strengthener, this exercise
requires flexibility. Start in the same
position as that described on the opposite
page, but place your bent leg in front
of your extended leg. Then lift. Be sure your
hips do not sag, your knee stays up and
your foot is flexed.

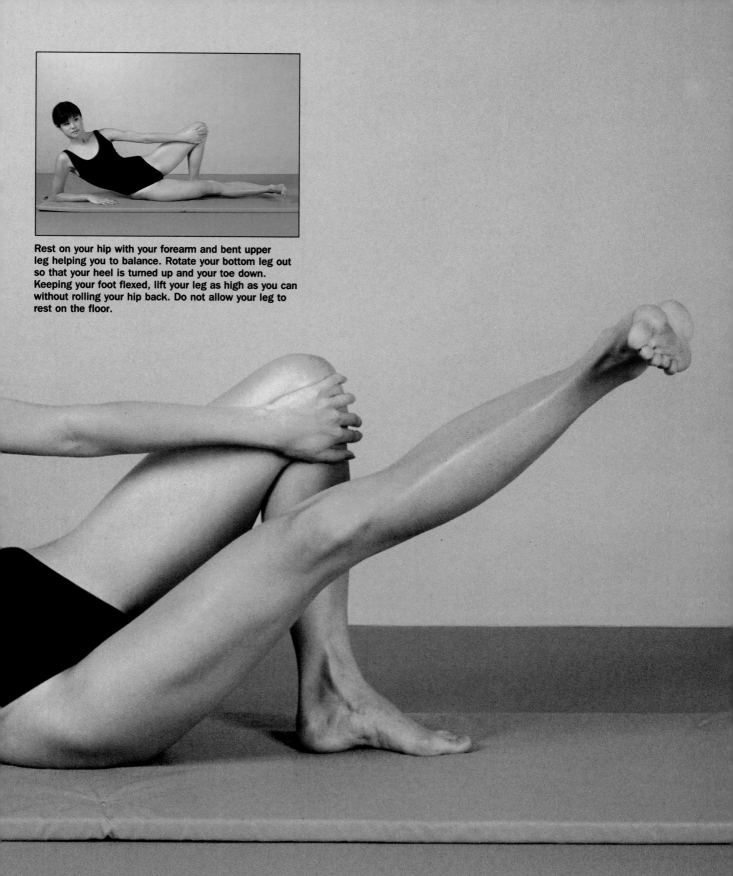

Rest on your hip with your forearm and bent upper leg helping you to balance. Rotate your bottom leg out so that your heel is turned up and your toe down. Keeping your foot flexed, lift your leg as high as you can without rolling your hip back. Do not allow your leg to rest on the floor.

Lower-Leg Shaping

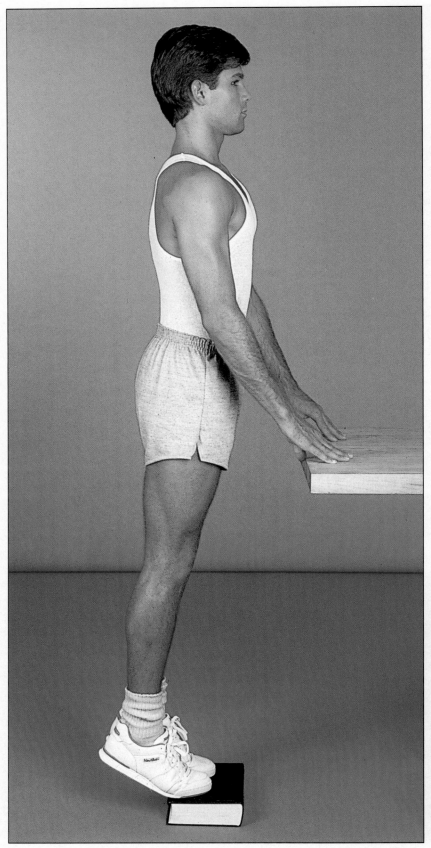

Stronger, shapelier calves are best built with calf lifts, which should always be done with your toes on a raised object like a book. This position prevents your calf muscles from shortening, which makes them more vulnerable to tearing. Balance calf lifts with the toe-tapping exercise below. This tones the muscles in the front of your lower leg and helps prevent the condition called shin splints, which often afflicts runners and those who do high-impact aerobic movement routines. In addition to strengthening the major calf muscles like the gastrocnemius and soleus, lower-leg work builds the muscles that control toe and foot movement and that subtly steer our bodies' direction.

With your toes pointed straight ahead, slowly rise on the balls of your feet, then lower your heels completely to the floor *(left)*. Use your hands only for balance, not support. Be sure that your ankles do not roll outward.

Sitting in a chair, lift the front of your foot as high as you can and tap your toe rhythmically to the floor at a rate of about one tap a second *(below)*. Continue for 30 to 60 seconds.

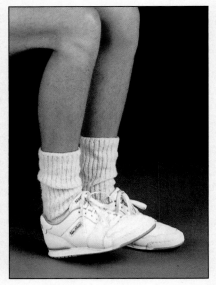

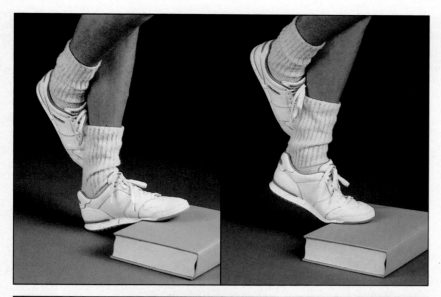

Intensify the effort by strengthening one calf at a time. Balance on the ball and toes of one foot with the other foot wrapped around the back of your ankle as you lift and lower. Do not pronate.

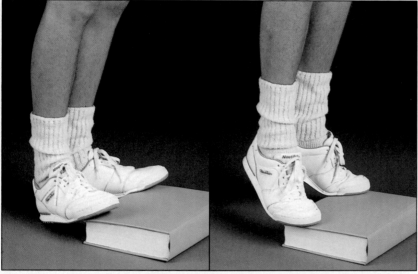

Lift with your heels together and toes pointed out to work major calf muscles and the outer peroneals, which help steady the leg and turn the foot out.

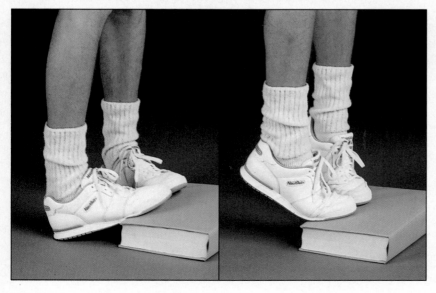

Do calf lifts with your toes together and your heels apart to add the inner tibeals to your workout. Strength in these muscles helps roll your feet in, enhancing agility as well as ankle stability.

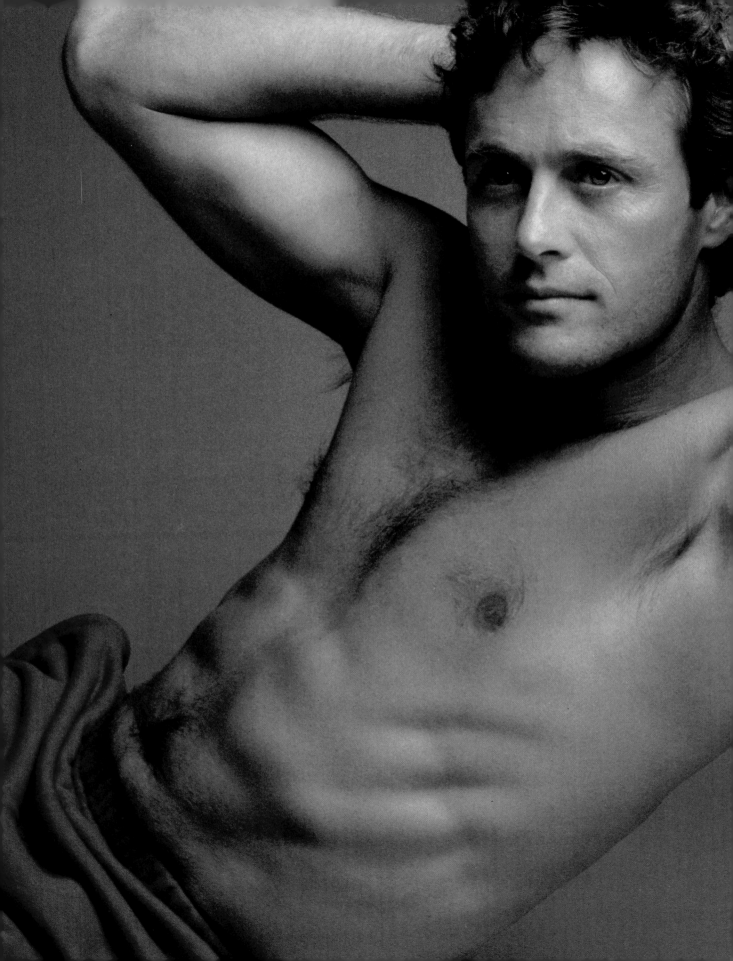

CHAPTER THREE

The Middle Body

*A flatter stomach and a stronger back
without strain*

Everyone wants a trim, toned waistline. Both men and women, according to one survey, express more concern about the shape of their midsections than about any other part of their body. For most of us, the concern may be purely esthetic. Taut, well-muscled middles look attractive. But this appeal also has a sound basis in physiology. A firm waist is generally considered an accurate signal of overall fitness.

The abdominal muscles are important to many everyday movements involving the torso. Walking, sitting, jumping, squatting, reaching — even breathing and good posture — depend on abdominals. These muscles stabilize or power your body in virtually every type of exercise, whether you are hitting a tennis shot or kicking a football. Like powerful rubber bands, the abdominals transfer force between your upper and lower body. Strong abdominal muscles make you a faster sprinter because your pumping arms help pull your legs into a burst of forward movement. And they mobilize force from your lower body that gives strength to upper body movements. Moreover, when working properly, they are like a natural girdle that supports both your organs and your back. You cannot have a healthy back or good posture without strong abdominals.

Unique among muscles, the abdominals control bones to which they are not attached. The rectus abdominis, for example, is a principal mover of your spine. Stretched between rib cage and pubic bone, this long muscle bends your spine forward and stabilizes the chest and abdomen in every movement. The rectus is also the muscle responsible for the "washboard" look seen in well-toned abdomens, an appearance caused by the tendinous bands that cross the muscle. It is the rectus that basically flattens the abdomen, though no one has a truly flat abdominal wall: Its curves accommodate internal organs. Because some exercises work the top of the rectus harder than the bottom — or the bottom harder than the top — thorough toning of the muscle requires exercises that involve both legs and upper body.

Assisting the rectus in flexing the spine are the external obliques, which also twist, turn and bend the middle body, and keep it erect. These sheetlike muscles overlap. On top, the external obliques wrap around your sides, coming to a V in front. Along the sides of your rib cage, they intersect sawtooth fashion with the serratus muscles. The serratus muscles help stabilize your rib cage when you breathe, but they get the most work from arm-raising exercises.

Underneath the externals, the internal obliques run diagonally opposite and form an upside-down V. All of the obliques are best developed by exercises that work your body at an angle, such as diagonal crunches *(pages 62-63)*.

Even the most well-exercised abdominals cannot tame a bulging belly area that is the site of excessive fat storage. If you are very overweight, these muscles, no matter how well toned, will remain hidden by fat stored below your skin. And pressure from fat stored internally will ensure that the muscles are stretched, making your abdomen protrude. To reduce fat here, as anywhere on the body, you have to diet and increase your caloric expenditure with aerobic exercise. But a protruding abdomen can also be the result of poor posture, which exaggerates any fat surplus and often contributes to backache as well. Toning your abdominal wall can help correct this condition by pulling your pelvis into better alignment and away from the common arched, swayback tilt or an overly forward thrust that is often associated with lower back pain. Your abdomen will appear flatter as well.

Of course, you also need to develop your back muscles for good posture and a pain-free back. The relevant muscles are primarily the erector spinae group, which runs along both sides of the spine from the base to the chest. This group consists of many intertwining, superficial muscles; none of them is very long or strong, but together they are crucial for good posture and for a back that does not ache.

Misconceptions abound about how to condition the hard-to-reach muscles of the middle body. For example, many people still regard the

Middle Body

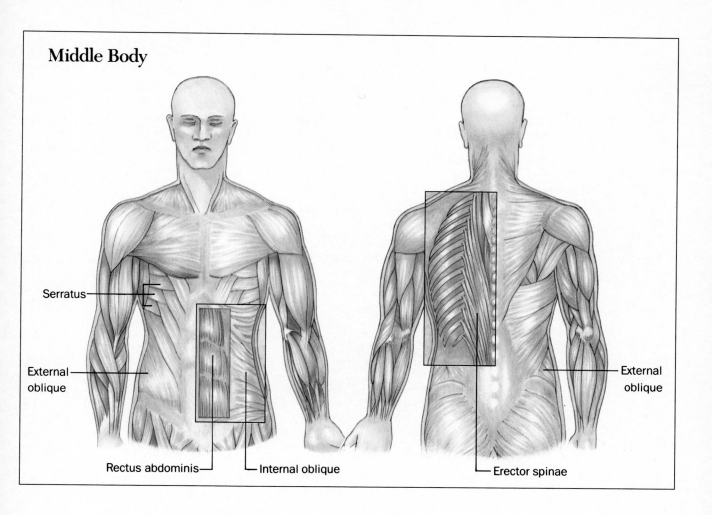

Serratus—

External—
oblique

External
oblique

Rectus abdominis—   — Internal oblique

Erector spinae

conventional bent-knee sit-up as the best all-around abdominal exercise. But as explained on page 60, the crunch, an alternative to the sit-up, is a safer and more effective exercise. Moreover, there is no "best" exercise, since no single movement can maximally engage all of the muscles involved in firming the midsection. In fact, more than one exercise is required simply to work the rectus abdominis thoroughly. In addition to the crunch, this chapter presents several crunch variations along with other abdominal exercises and a special program of exercises for the back.

When doing these exercises, inhale during the relaxed phase and exhale during the exertion (which should allow you to pull your abdomen in). You can also try breathing in your upper chest, using rapid puffs, when abdominal work grows intense. Work the muscles through their full range of motion in each exercise, though this movement may be small in certain positions. Not returning completely to a rest position will help keep tension in the muscles throughout the exercise. And rather than let gravity pull you quickly back to earth, roll down as slowly as possible. This will also help protect your back from strain. Be sure to balance your abdominal work with back-strengthening exercises.

Warm-Ups

The routine on these two pages not only readies the abdominal muscles for exercise, but also releases tension around the spine, an area that is often difficult to relax and vulnerable to strain. In this way, the warm-up helps ensure safety when you exert yourself in the toning exercises that follow. An added benefit of the routine is a healthful massage to internal organs.

This set contains warming and limbering movements. It is not necessary to stretch the abdominal muscles themselves. They are stretched daily as you sit, stand, move about and breathe.

If you have not already warmed up, first jog in place for several minutes or perform some other aerobic activity (like an aerobic dance routine or riding a stationary bicycle).

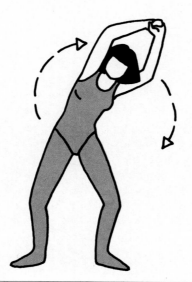

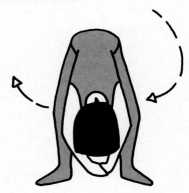

Clasp your hands over your head and bend your knees. Moving from your waist and hip joint, make big, easy circles with your arms and torso. Do 10 circles right, then 10 more circles left.

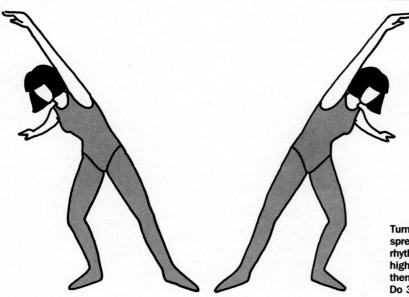

Turn your feet out in a wide stance and spread your arms. Lunge and twist rhythmically from right to left, reaching up high with your right arm as you turn left, then up with your left arm as you turn right. Do 30 complete turns.

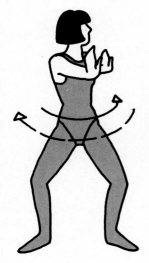

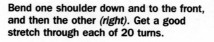

Rotate only your upper body from the waist as you swing from side to side 20 times with your arms outstretched and hands flexed (left). Keep your knees bent and pelvis facing front.

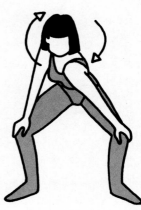

Bend one shoulder down and to the front, and then the other (right). Get a good stretch through each of 20 turns.

The Crunch

The crunch is the most efficient and the safest way to tone abdominal muscles. This exercise focuses effort on the crucial layer of muscle covering your midsection from rib cage to pubic bone. It bypasses muscles that may well be strong enough already, like hip flexors. It avoids stressing the small of the back, which can happen when your back arches as you rise. And if done correctly, without jerking the neck, the crunch protects you from upper cervical strain as well.

All of these reasons make the crunch superior to the sit-up when the sit-up involves a lift of more than 45 degrees from the floor — the level at which scientists have determined that hip-flexor involvement occurs. Holding your feet down does not help. This only emphasizes the hip flexors and detracts from the work of the abdominals. And if you do the sit-up with your legs straight, you risk lower back strain.

Technique is everything with crunches. The results you get will depend not on how many you do, but how well you do them. Start with one of the crunches for the rectus and one diagonal crunch, done left and right, for your obliques. Beginners or people with back problems should work the elevated crunches on pages 64-65 for both muscles.

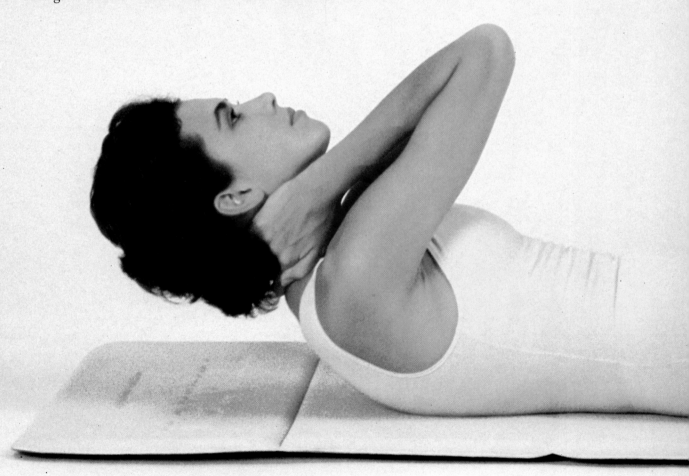

To perform the basic crunch, shown below, lie with your back flat on the floor and your legs comfortably drawn up to about a 90-degree angle. Support the back of your neck just below your skull with your hands. Point elbows forward. Slowly lift your upper body with your abdominal muscles, raising yourself no higher than the bottom of your shoulder blades. Let the weight of your head hang, supported by your hands. Use alternative arm positions to vary the amount of effort. For the least effort, reach your arms forward *(top right)*. Add exertion by folding your arms across your chest *(middle right)*. Or spread your elbows, placing your hands behind your head for more difficulty *(bottom right)*. When using alternative arm positions, be sure not to jerk your neck up as you lift.

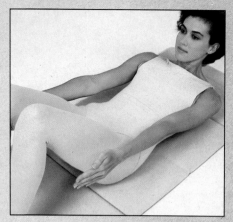

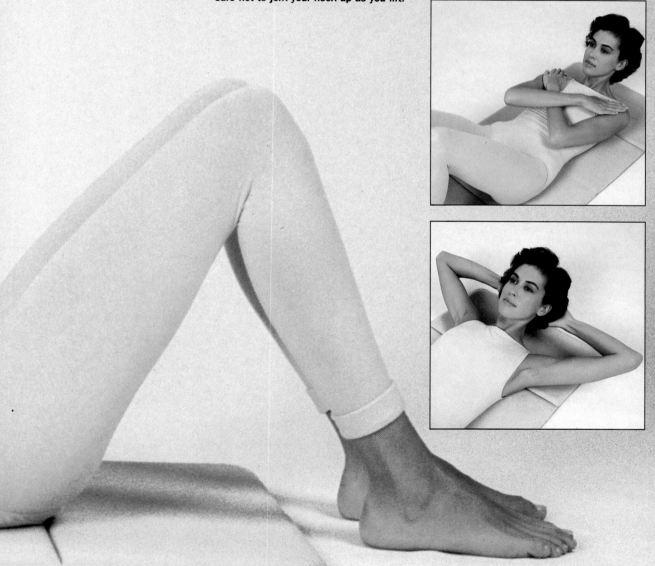

The Diagonal Crunch

To tone the muscles that shape the sides of your waist and provide the power for torso twists and turns, you must pull across your abdomen as if tightening an X-shaped band, one crosspiece at a time. This enlists your obliques to their maximum.

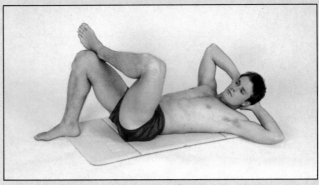

Start with your head and shoulder slightly raised *(above)* and twist your elbow toward your knee *(below)*. Complete sets for one side of your torso before switching to the other side.

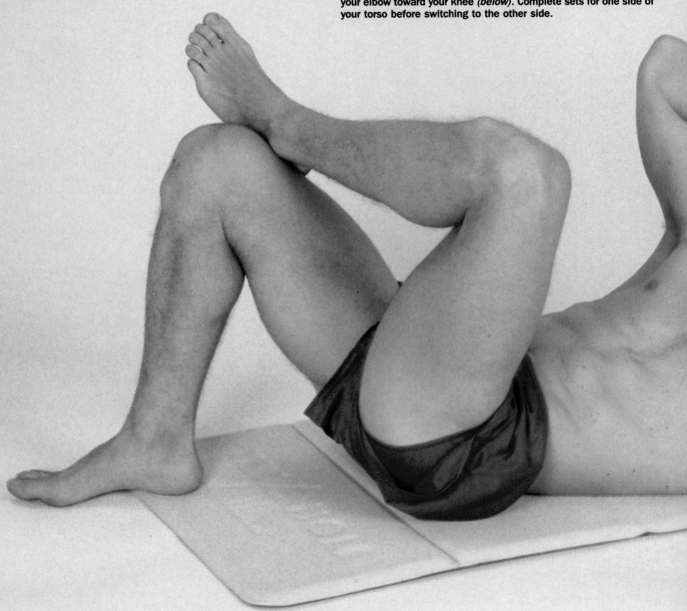

THESE TWO COUPLES HAVE IDENTICAL ACCOMMODATIONS ON THE SAME CRUISE...
YET:

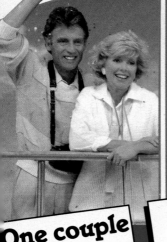

One couple paid
$1,095 per person

One couple paid
$489 per person

because they are members of the

SEARS DISCOUNT TRAVEL CLUB

(They have all the status and privileges of full-fare passengers...because nobody knows they paid 53% less)

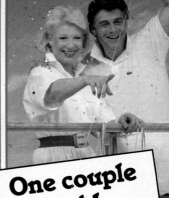

NOW!
YOU CAN TRAVEL ANYWHERE...

SEARS SHOP at HOME SERVICE

BY MAIL OR PHONE ONLY
Not available in Sears retail stores or catalog
(Use order form inside)

OR LOOK AT THESE OTHER FANTASTIC BARGAINS!

Some more examples of recent Sears Discount Travel Club trips:

FOLD ▶

COMPLETE VACATIONS

4 days, 3 nights Las Vegas

Regular Price **Club Price**

Includes round-trip air fare from Chicago, and hotel

SAVE 63% . . . . ~~$274~~ **$99**

8 days, 7 nights Jamaica

Includes round-trip air fare from Chicago, and 7 nights at Toby Inn

SAVE 57% . . . . ~~$459~~ **$199**

CRUISES

7 nights Caribbean Cruise

Includes round-trip air fare from 140 cities to Miami

SAVE 53% . . . . ~~$1,095~~ **$489**

7 nights Bermuda Cruise

New York to Bermuda

SAVE 52% . . . . ~~$1,095~~ **$529**

ROUND-TRIP AIR ONLY

New York to London

7 nights

SAVE 37% . . . . ~~$638~~ **$399**

Detroit to Las Vegas

SAVE 65% . . . . ~~$199~~ **$69**

FOI

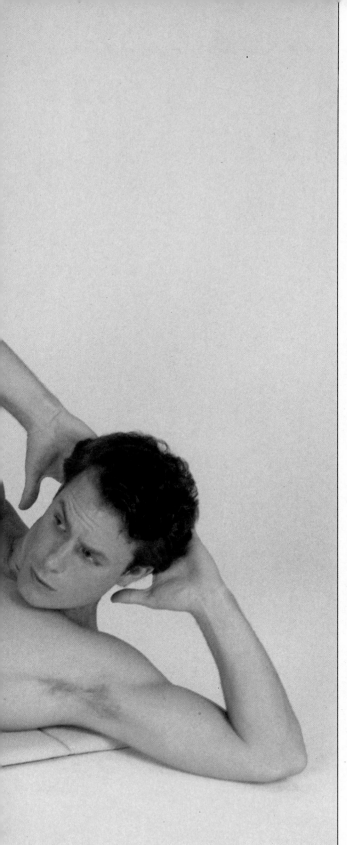

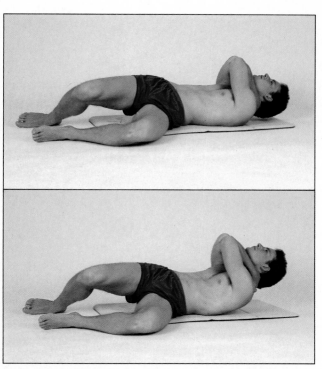

Support your neck by placing your hands at the base of your skull. Bend your legs, letting them flop to the left, the bottom one resting on the floor *(top)*. Lift, letting your head hang *(bottom)*.

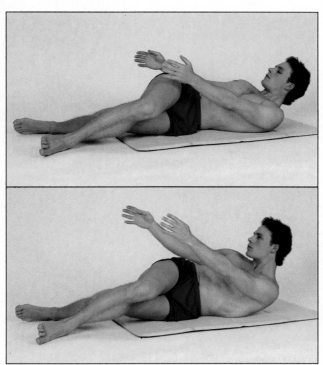

Intensify diagonals by lying on one hip with your bent legs crossed to the side. Begin with your head and shoulders slightly lifted, arms reaching out *(top)*. Continue reaching as you roll up slowly *(bottom)*. Never roll all the way down.

63

The Elevated Crunch

If you have back trouble or especially weak abdominal muscles, safeguard your back by performing crunches with your legs raised and supported. Beginners should start with elevated crunches, too. This position keeps your lower back securely on the floor and defeats any attempt to use hip flexors rather than abdominals. You may use any bench, chair or sofa of the right height. Do the basic version, shown on the opposite page, to work the rectus abdominis or the variation shown below to work the obliques.

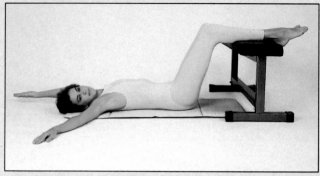

To work your obliques, lie on your back with your bent legs resting on a stable support and your arms raised to form a wide V over your head *(above)*. Lift your left arm slowly and reach across your torso to the right of your knees *(below)*. Do all the sets on that side before switching to your right arm.

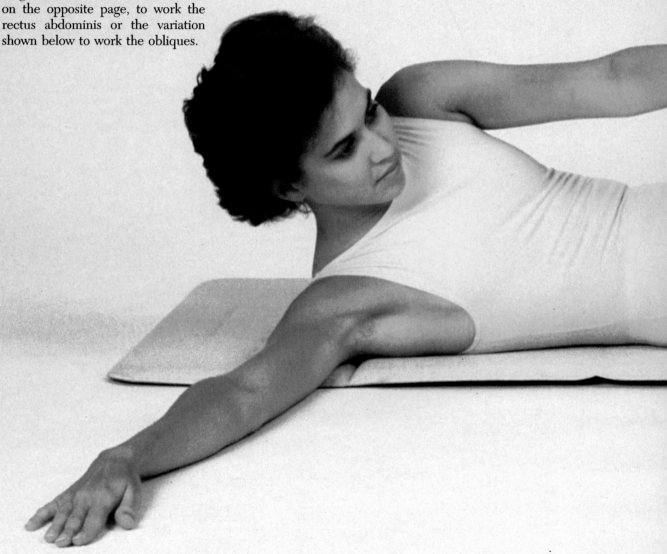

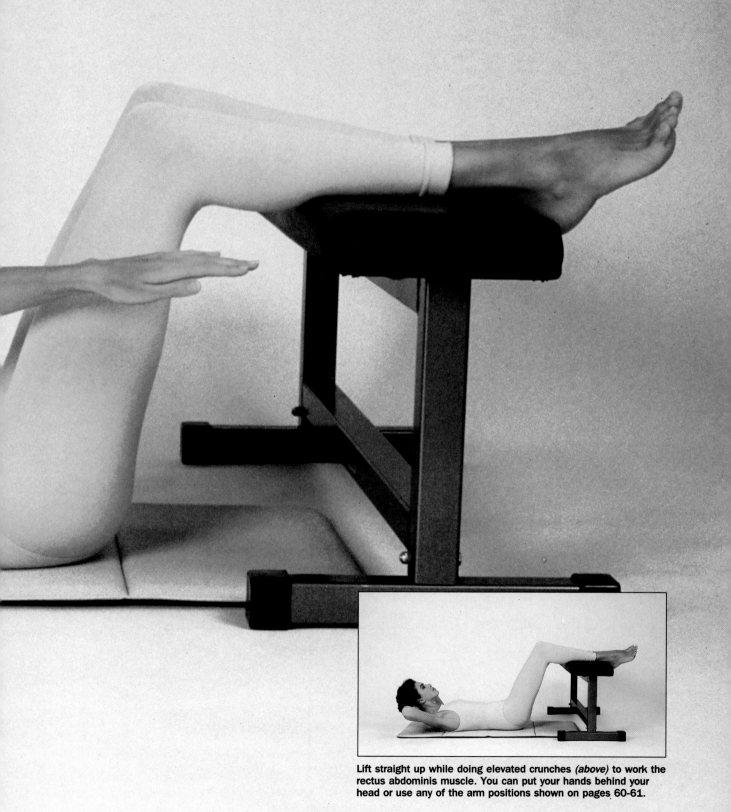

Lift straight up while doing elevated crunches *(above)* to work the rectus abdominis muscle. You can put your hands behind your head or use any of the arm positions shown on pages 60-61.

The Diamond Crunch

If your torso is long or your back inflexible, this will help you focus on abdominals and avoid exercising hip flexors. Put the soles of your feet together and spread your bent legs. Support your head with your hands *(below)*. Contract your abdominals and lift *(bottom)*. Do not jerk your head forward.

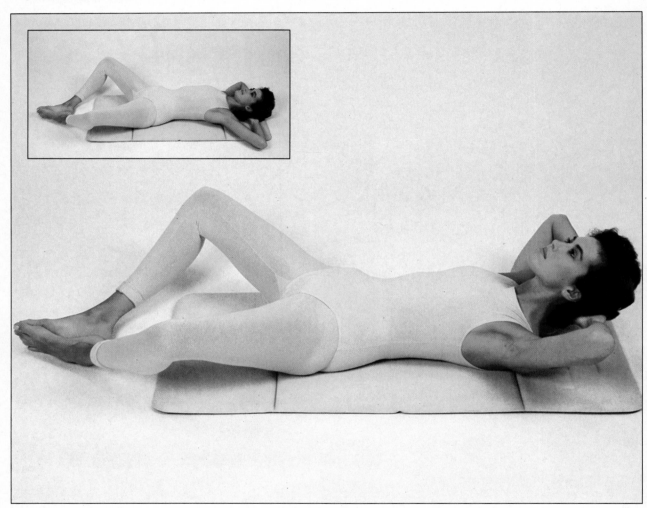

The Hip Lift

Do this exercise for the lower rectus on your back with your legs raised and ankles crossed, your head lifted and supported by your hands *(opposite)*. Contract your lower abdominals to raise your hips slightly off the floor.

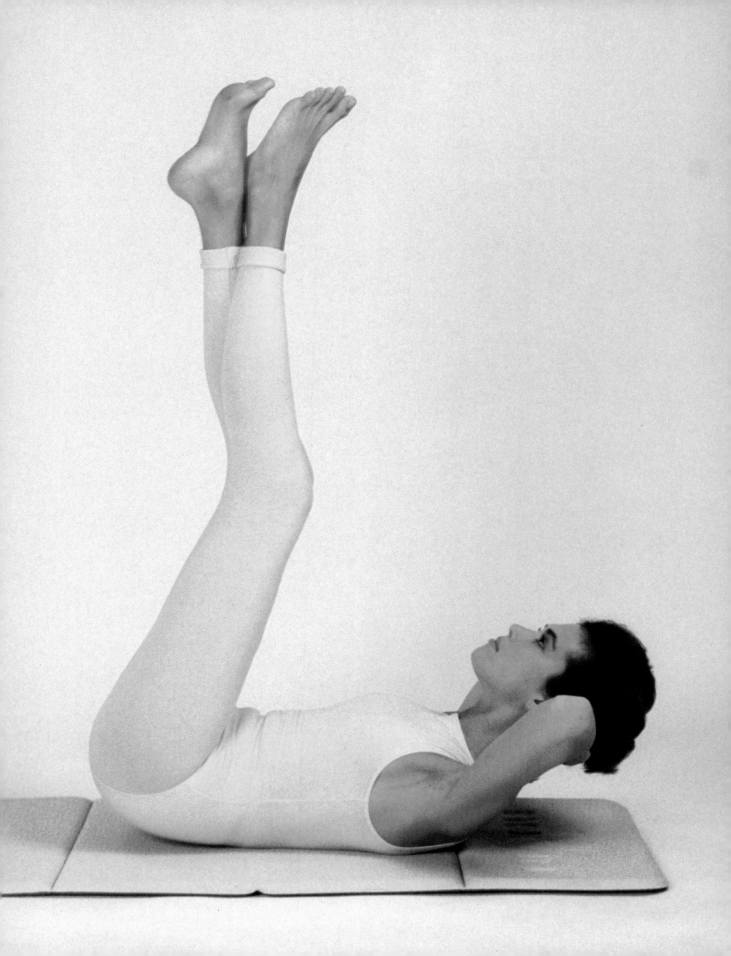

The Negative Sit-Up

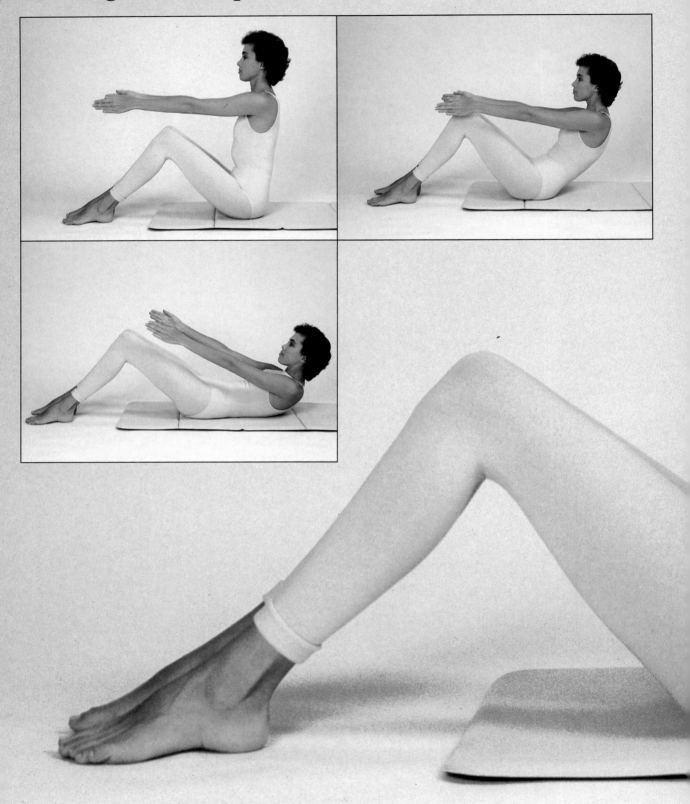

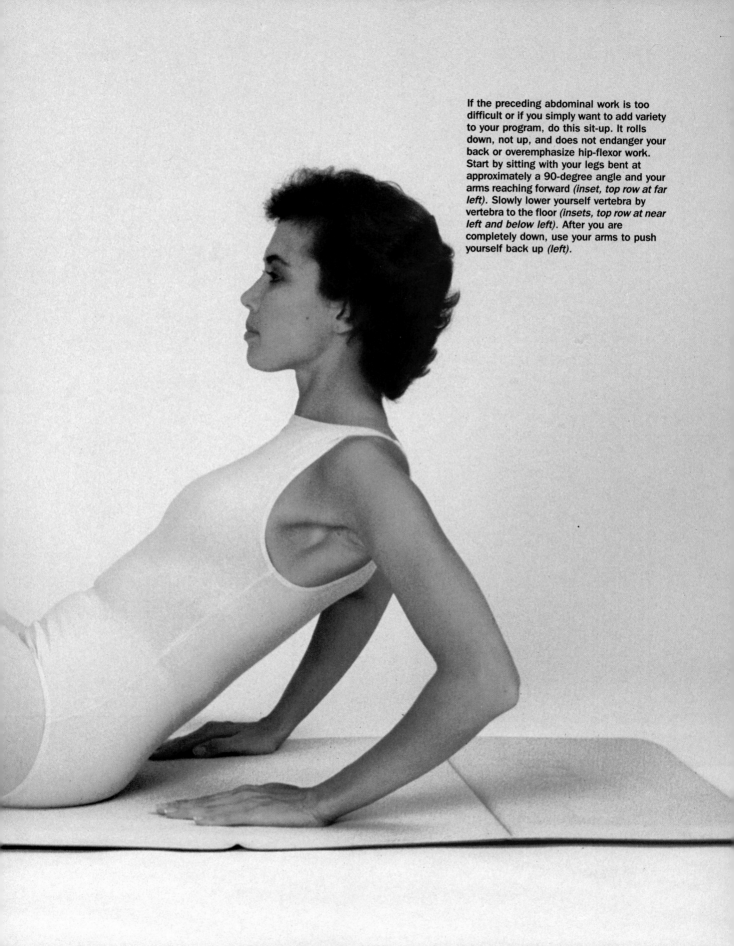

If the preceding abdominal work is too difficult or if you simply want to add variety to your program, do this sit-up. It rolls down, not up, and does not endanger your back or overemphasize hip-flexor work. Start by sitting with your legs bent at approximately a 90-degree angle and your arms reaching forward *(inset, top row at far left)*. Slowly lower yourself vertebra by vertebra to the floor *(insets, top row at near left and below left)*. After you are completely down, use your arms to push yourself back up *(left)*.

The Bicycle

These versions of the bicycle effectively stress both upper and lower abdominals simultaneously. In addition, they work both the rectus and the obliques. Any of the three degrees of difficulty shown can provide a thorough abdominal workout. Attempt the intermediate and advanced versions only if you can do them without lifting your lower back from the floor. Try the intermediate once you can do three sets of 20 in the beginning position. Move on to the advanced version when you can do three sets of the intermediate.

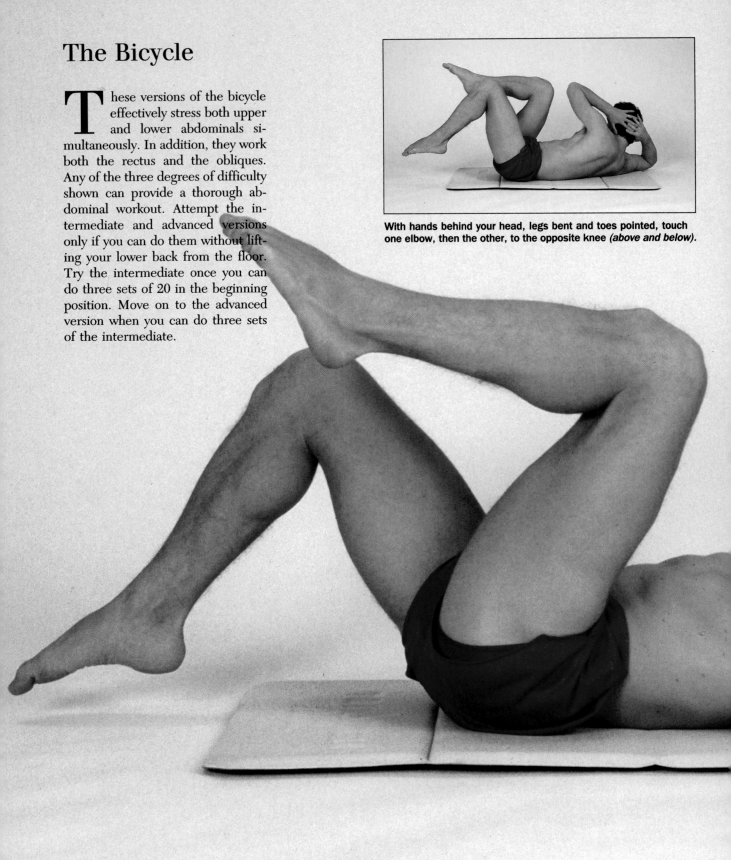

With hands behind your head, legs bent and toes pointed, touch one elbow, then the other, to the opposite knee *(above and below)*.

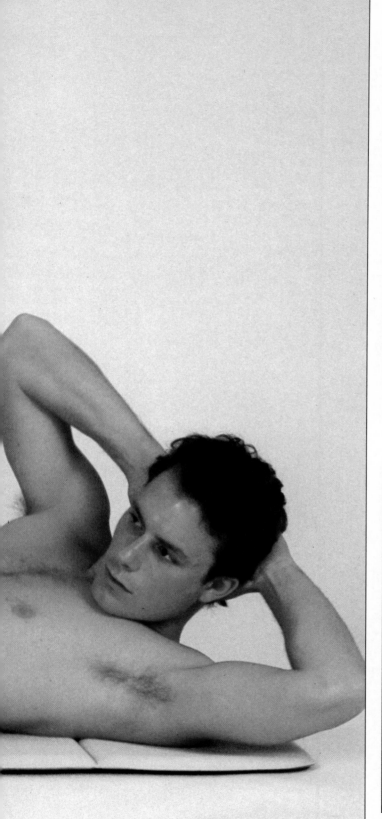

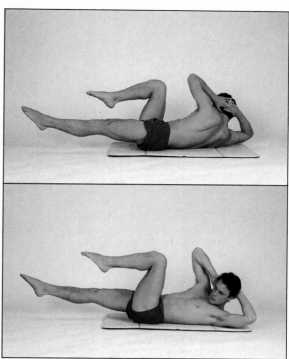

To do the intermediate version, fully extend each leg in turn after you pull your knee in toward its opposing elbow *(above)*.

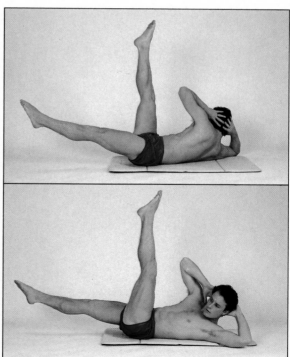

Do the advanced version with legs straight and toes pointed. Alternately bend one leg at the hip and then the other, drawing each leg toward the opposing elbow *(above)*.

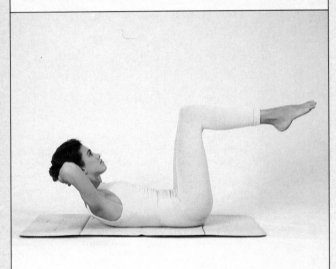

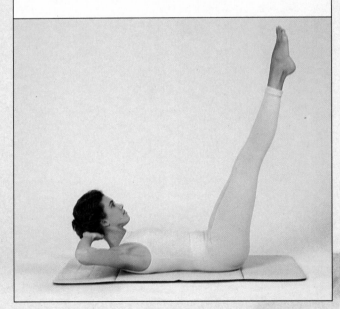

The V-Up

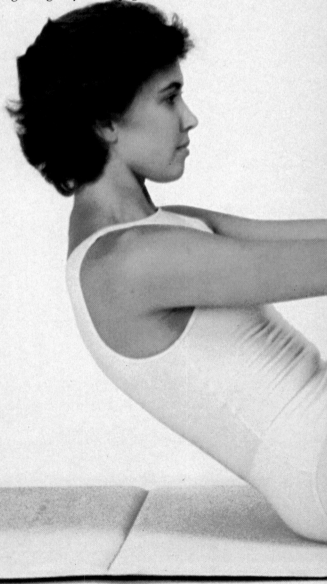

A classic exercise, the properly performed V-up targets the lower abdominals. Many other V-ups require leg lifts. These V-ups, however, start with legs raised to avoid engaging the hip flexors. Because they do not require you to jerk your legs into the air as do standard V-ups, they are also safer for your back. If you have a weak back or feel back strain, however, choose an easier exercise like the beginning bicycle on pages 70-71.

To do the beginning V-up, lie flat on your back, hands behind your head, your legs bent at a right angle *(top)*. Lift your head and shoulders *(middle)*. Straighten your legs and point your toes *(bottom)*.

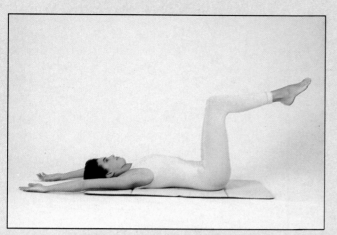

Start the intermediate V-up on your back with hands stretched behind your head, your bent legs held at an angle of about 90 degrees *(above)*. Bring your arms over your head, raise your upper body and reach your hands beyond your knees, parallel with lower legs *(below)*.

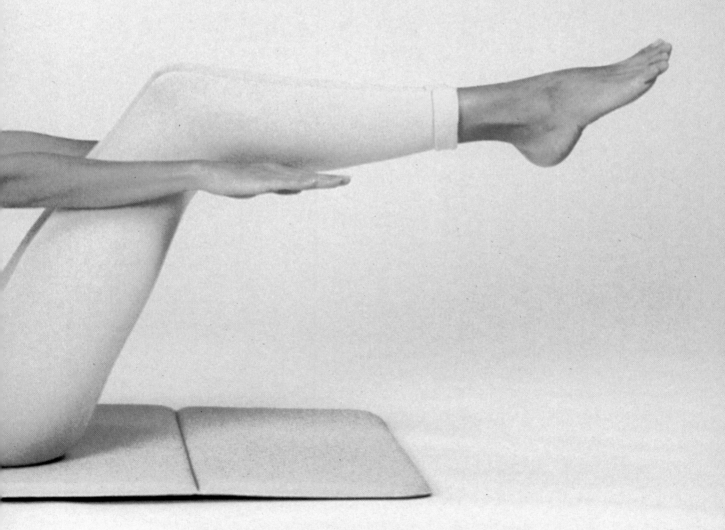

The Advanced V-Up

This challenging exercise tightens and tones both upper and lower abdominals. It also helps work your shoulders, chest and back. And it can advance the development of balance and grace as it firms your midsection. Designed to avoid putting stress on the lower back, this is still a demanding exercise. You should thoroughly master the intermediate V-up before attempting this version. If you feel any discomfort in your back, return to an easier version.

People who have tight lower backs may not find the V-up comfortable no matter how well developed their abdominal muscles are. They will get more benefits and more enjoyment from exercises providing continuous back support. The bicycle on pages 70-71, particularly the beginning and intermediate, can help them work their lower abdominals.

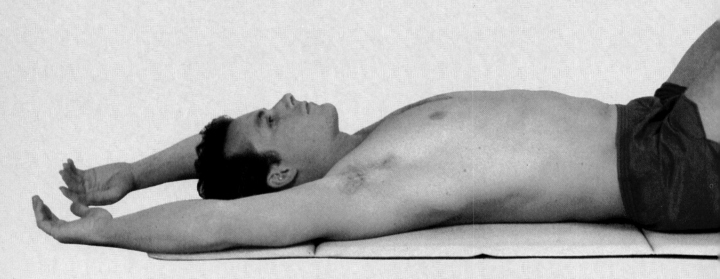

Lie with your back flat on the floor, your arms over your head and your legs raised at about a 45-degree angle *(above)*. Using your abdominal muscles, reach over and pull your upper body into a V with your legs, stretching your fingers toward your toes *(opposite)*.

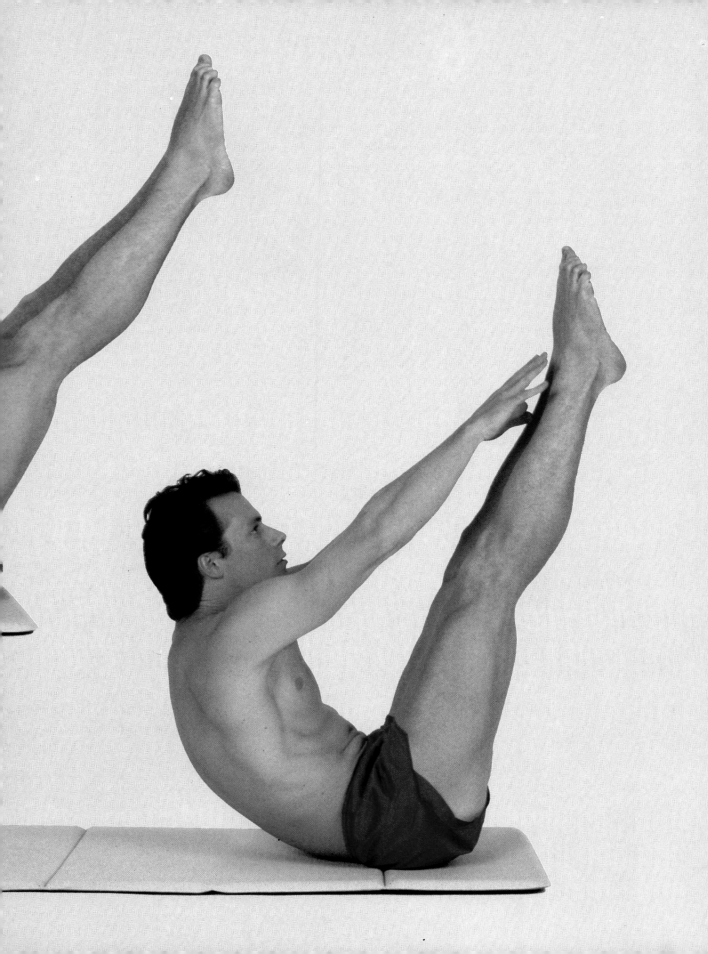

Back Strength

Because strong abdominals should be balanced by a strong back, your midsection program should include work to develop the erector spinae muscle group. (However, if you suffer back pain, consult your doctor before doing these strength exercises.) Start by sitting on the edge of a weight bench or chair. Put your hands behind your head and bend forward *(inset)*. Lift up slowly to about a 45-degree angle but do not go any higher *(right)*.

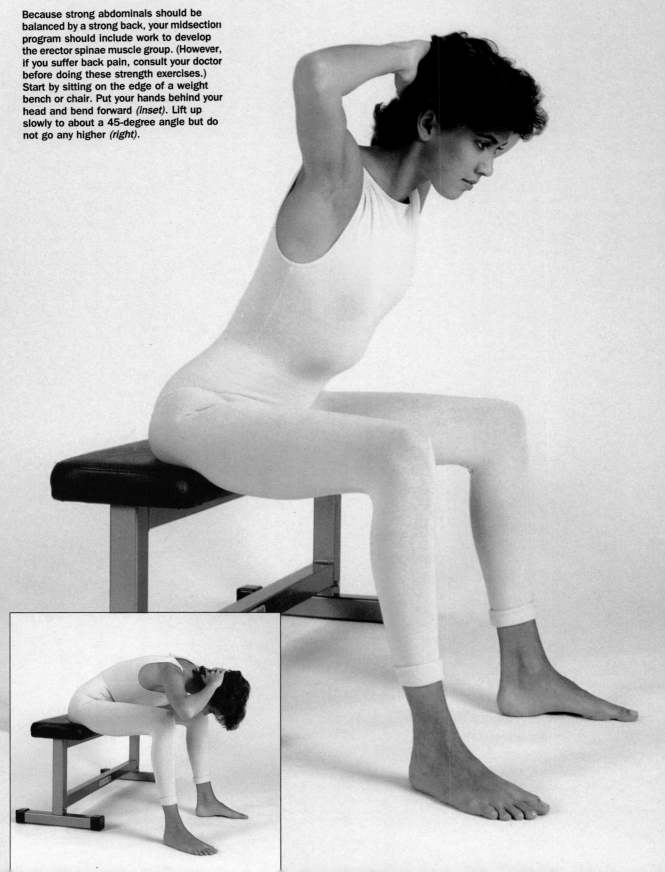

Lie face down on a weight bench or sturdy table, your hands behind your head, with the top of your chest over the edge *(right)*. If you are on a table, use a folded towel for padding. Lift your upper body until you are about parallel to the floor *(below)*.

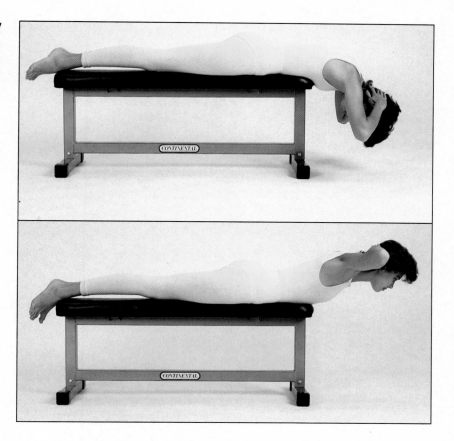

Lie stomach down on a weight bench or heavy table with your head lifted. Hang your bent legs over the end of the bench from the hip joint. Hold onto the bench for support *(right)*. Then extend your legs and point your toes until you are parallel to the floor or a little higher *(below)*.

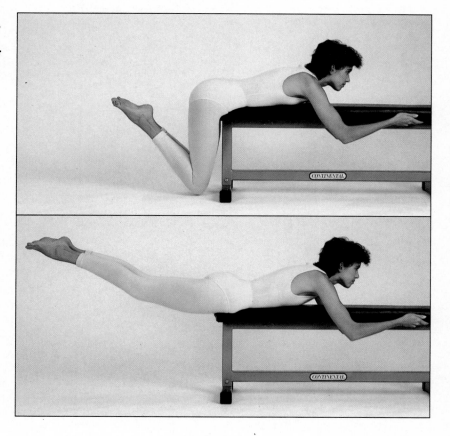

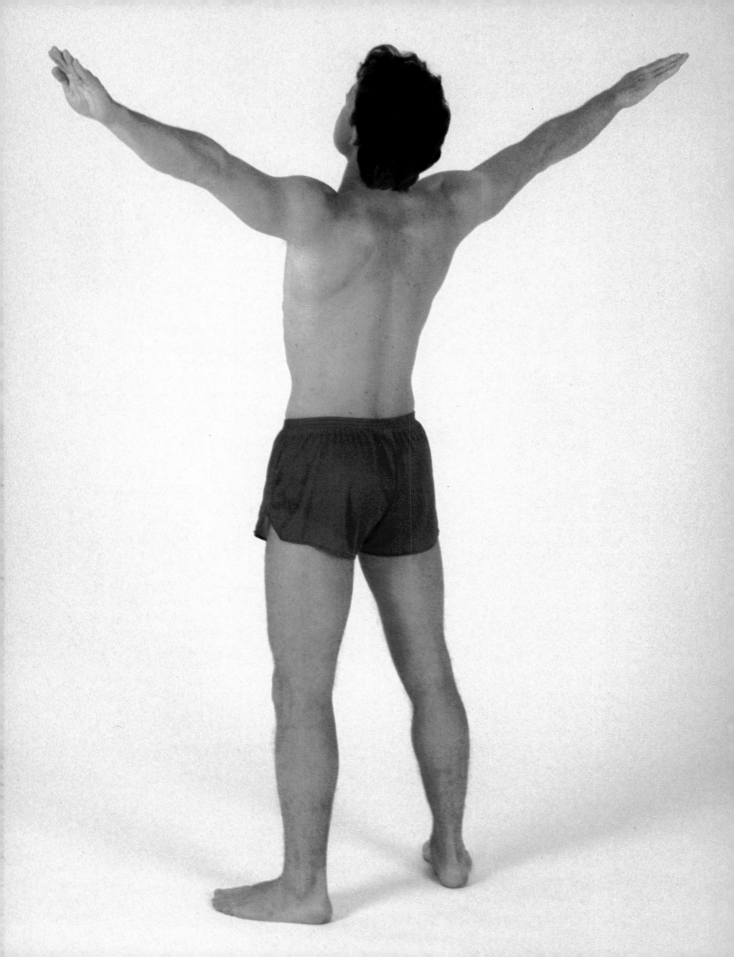

The Good-Back Program

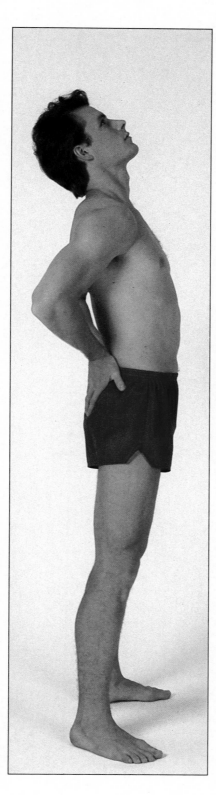

Though they are vital, strong abdominal and back muscles together cannot give you all the protection you need against common causes of back strain, including poor posture. Adding a few simple exercises to your program can help you avoid the back pain that afflicts an estimated 80 percent of adults.

The exercises in this section help counteract problems created by too strong or too tight hip flexors, which join your pelvis and your spine to your thighbones. Leg exercises such as running, bicycling and walking build strong hip flexors that pull up on the back of the pelvis. If not resisted, the pelvis tilts forward, overstressing muscles in the lumbar spine region. The result: muscle strain, spasm and ache. In addition, your abdomen protrudes, putting more strain on the small of your back.

Counteracting this problem calls for loosening hip flexors along with strengthening abdominals and back muscles. The final important step is to train the muscles that support your pelvis to assume the correct tilt. This helps ensure good posture and avoid a lumbar-stressing swayback.

These exercises are designed not only to prevent back trouble, but to help relieve stiffness or soreness in your back without overtaxing weak muscles. However, if you suffer back discomfort, consult a doctor before beginning this program.

Except for the final three, which are back strengtheners and which you should work up to, the exercises may be done as frequently as you wish, no matter what your level of fitness. If you care to do more repetitions or longer holds than suggested, that, too, is fine.

Begin to warm your back with this soaring reach *(opposite)*. Stand with your feet shoulder width apart, so that your weight is distributed evenly. Reach up and back, spreading your arms like wings. Lift your face. Keep your hips right below your rib cage. Breathe in and out deeply 10 times.

Align your pelvis properly *(right)*. Stand at ease. Rest your hands on the small of your back. Lift the top of your chest, raise your chin and keep your hips directly below your rib cage. Hold this pose one minute, breathing normally. This position eases the strain on your back.

Knee Press

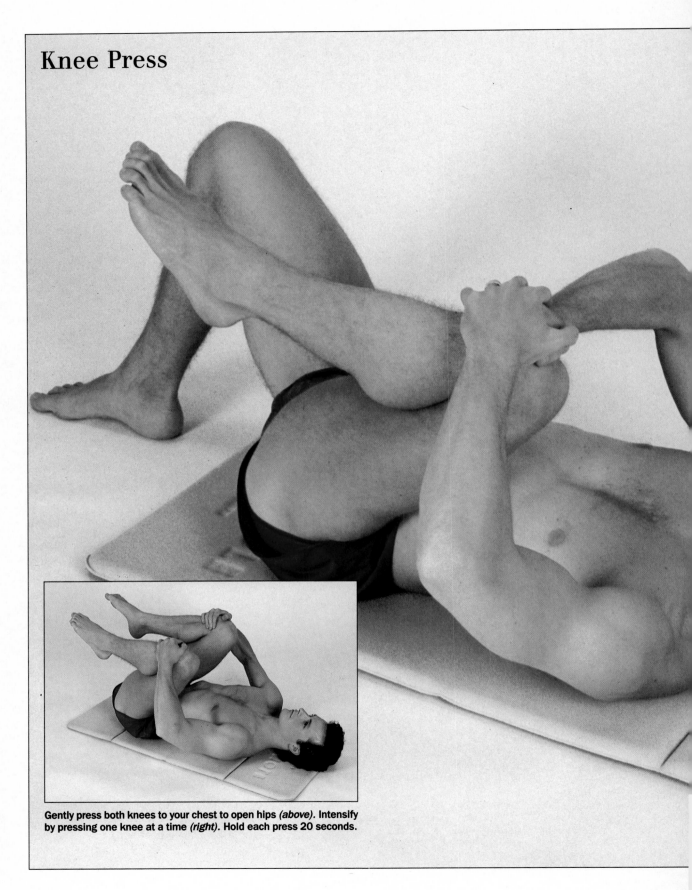

Gently press both knees to your chest to open hips *(above)***. Intensify by pressing one knee at a time** *(right)***. Hold each press 20 seconds.**

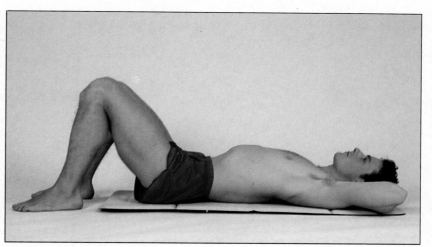

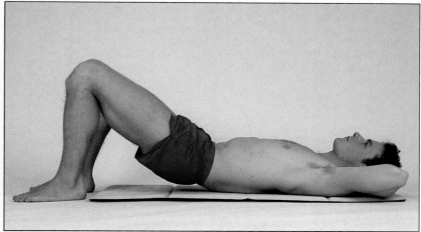

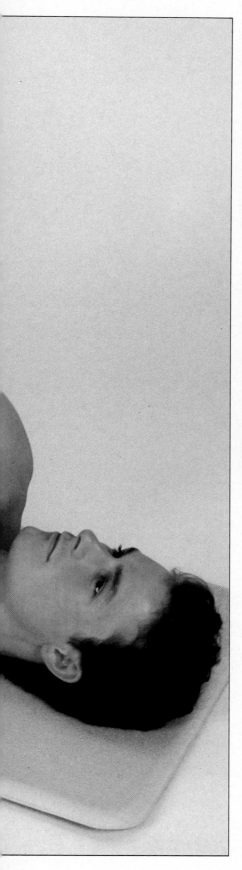

Pelvic Tilt

Place your hands comfortably under your head. Bend your legs up, rest your feet on the floor and flatten your lower back *(top)*. Then slowly roll your hips up until you reach your waistline *(above)*. Feel your lower spine lengthen as your pelvis tilts. Hold for 10 seconds, then slowly roll back down. Repeat three times.

Cobra and Sphinx

To perform the cobra, place your hands under your shoulders and slowly raise your upper body *(above)*. Use the muscles along your spine as well as the strength of your arms. Rise as high as you can without experiencing discomfort. Keep your head up, your elbows bent and your shoulders down *(right)*. Hold for 10 seconds or longer.

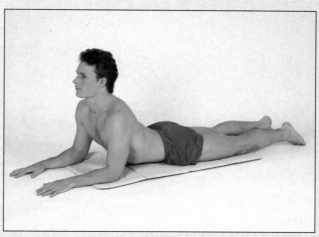

If the cobra is too difficult, do the sphinx *(above)*. **Lie face down with your arms bent by your sides. Lift your head and chest as you slide your forearms up until your elbows are directly below your shoulders. (It should feel as if there were a string lifting the top of your head toward the ceiling.) Do not hunch your shoulders. Hold for at least 10 seconds.**

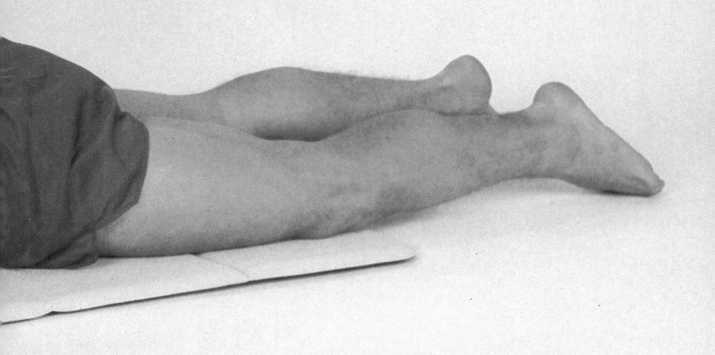

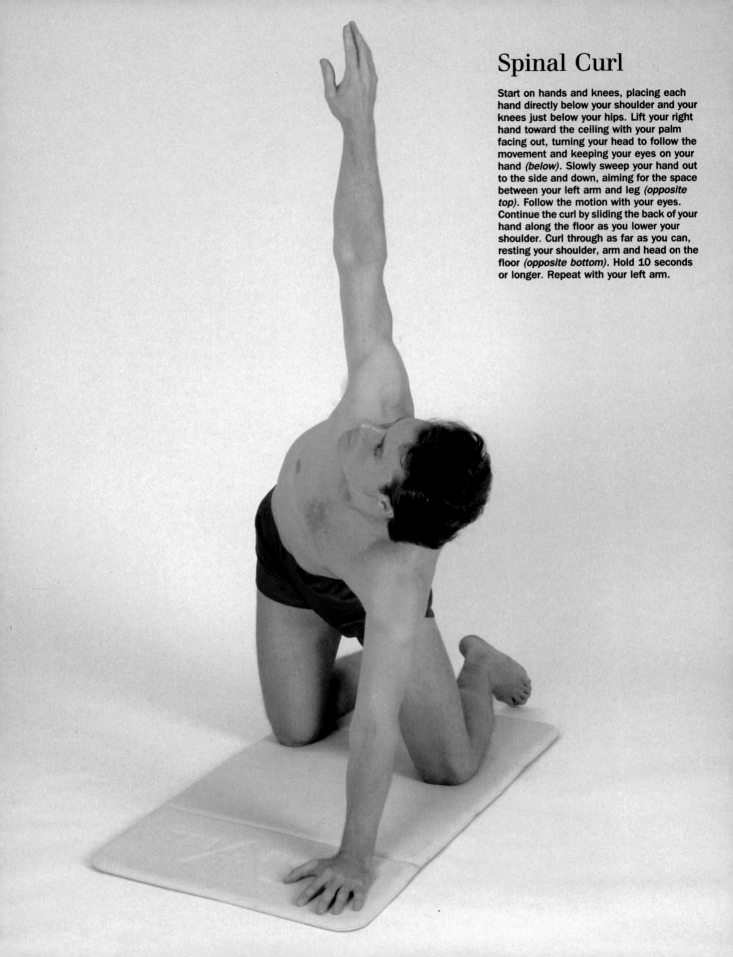

Spinal Curl

Start on hands and knees, placing each hand directly below your shoulder and your knees just below your hips. Lift your right hand toward the ceiling with your palm facing out, turning your head to follow the movement and keeping your eyes on your hand *(below)*. Slowly sweep your hand out to the side and down, aiming for the space between your left arm and leg *(opposite top)*. Follow the motion with your eyes. Continue the curl by sliding the back of your hand along the floor as you lower your shoulder. Curl through as far as you can, resting your shoulder, arm and head on the floor *(opposite bottom)*. Hold 10 seconds or longer. Repeat with your left arm.

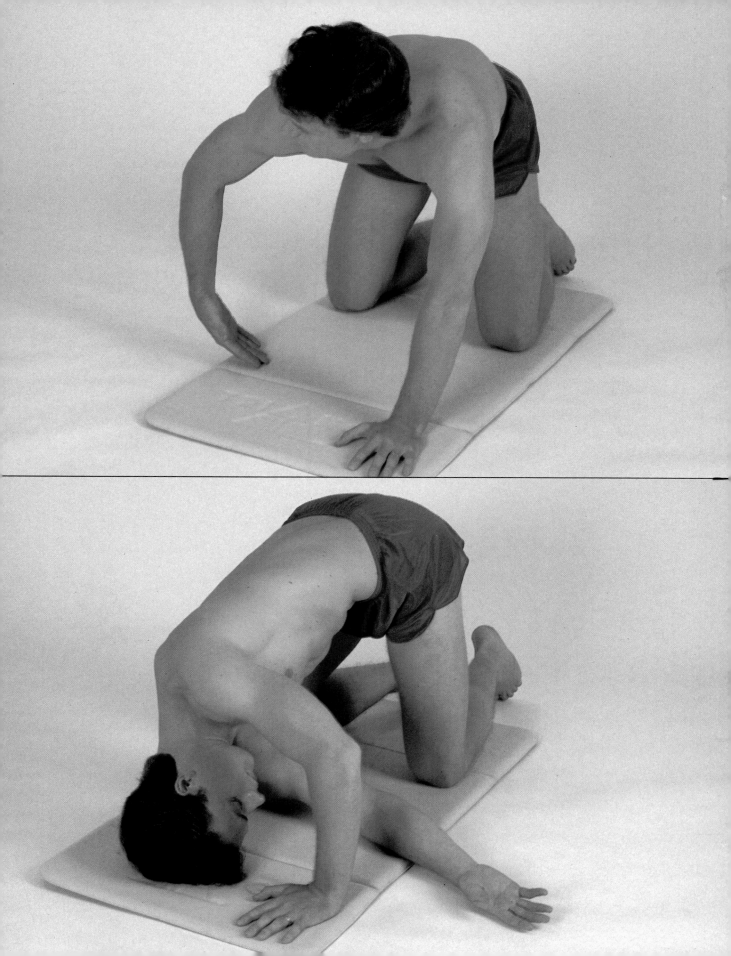

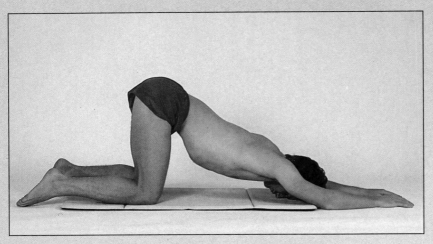

The Child

Rest your forehead on a mat or rug, stretch your arms out in front of you and lift your hips so that your bent knees support most of your weight *(left)*. Relax your back completely. Remain in this posture for half a minute. Then let your upper body slide toward your knees as your hips sink onto your lower legs *(below)*. Stay in this pose as long as you wish, letting all the tension in your body evaporate.

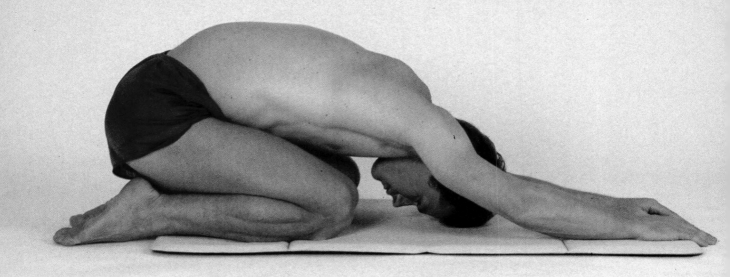

The Cat

Assume a catlike position with your hands beneath your shoulders and your knees under your hips *(right)*. Bend your spine down so that your rib cage sinks, your pelvis tilts toward your legs and the top of your head rises. Hold for a count of five. Then arch your spine, bending your head down and drawing your abdomen in as far as you can *(below)*. Hold for another five count. Repeat this sequence twice.

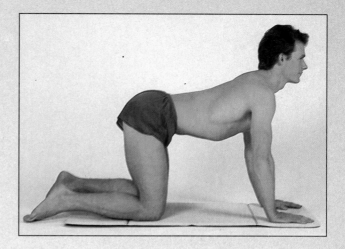

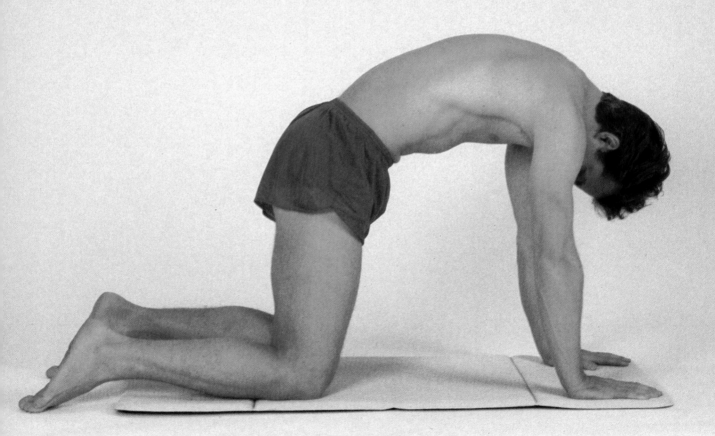

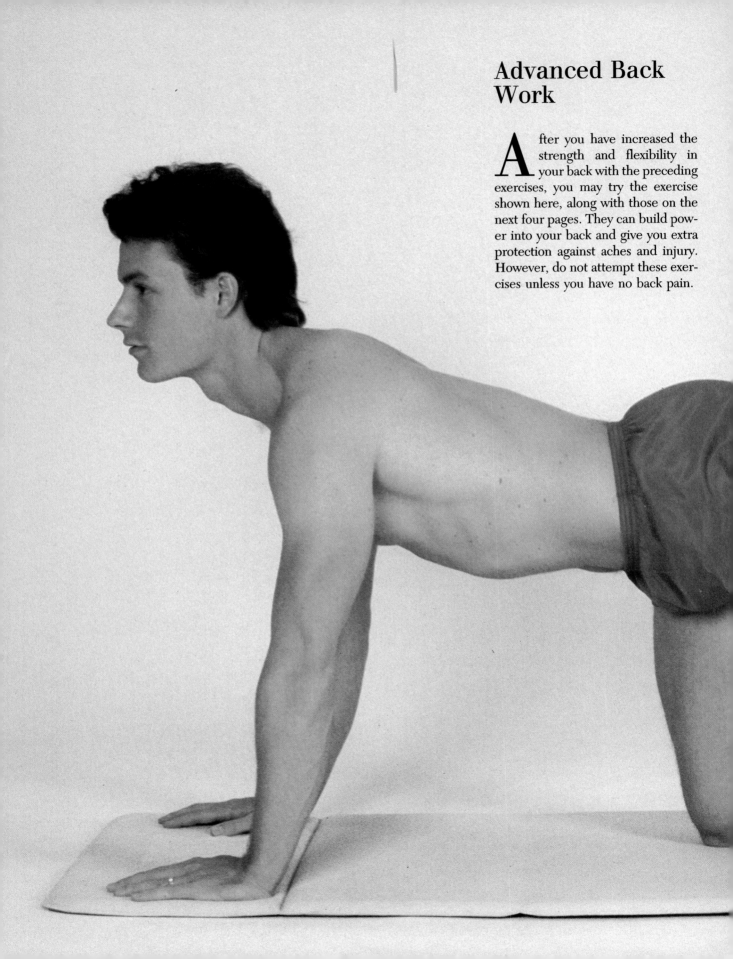

Advanced Back Work

After you have increased the strength and flexibility in your back with the preceding exercises, you may try the exercise shown here, along with those on the next four pages. They can build power into your back and give you extra protection against aches and injury. However, do not attempt these exercises unless you have no back pain.

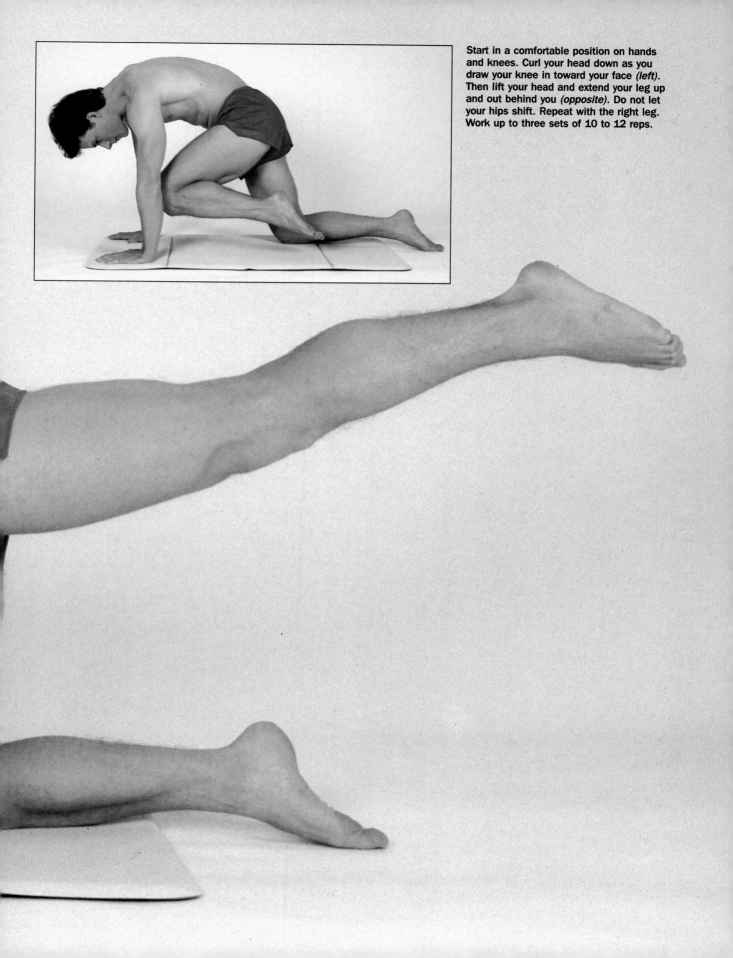

Start in a comfortable position on hands and knees. Curl your head down as you draw your knee in toward your face *(left)*. Then lift your head and extend your leg up and out behind you *(opposite)*. Do not let your hips shift. Repeat with the right leg. Work up to three sets of 10 to 12 reps.

Back Diagonal

Begin on all fours with knees below hips and hands below shoulders *(right)*. Without shifting your torso, reach forward with your right hand and point your left foot to the rear. Do not let your hip or shoulder sag, move forward or move back *(below)*. Return to the starting position. Reach forward with your left hand and point back with your right toe, maintaining the same posture *(inset opposite)*. Work up to three sets of 10 repetitions of this sequence.

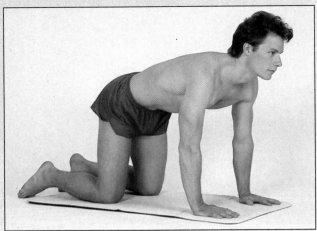

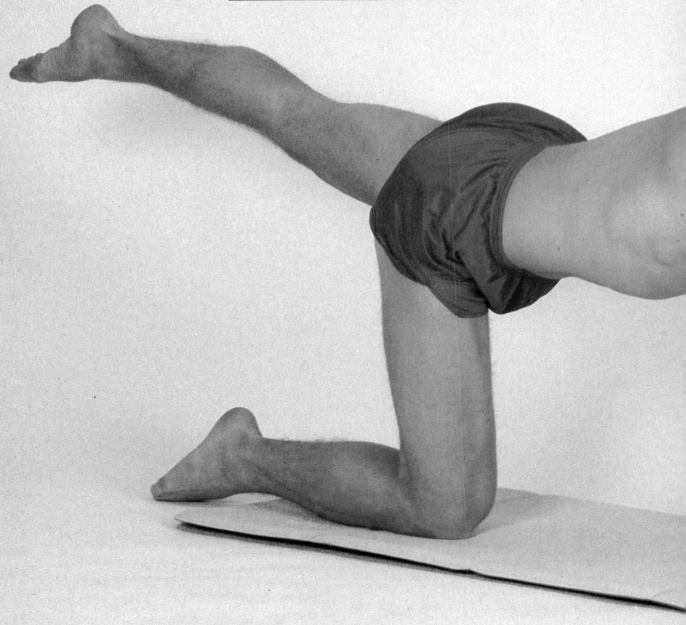

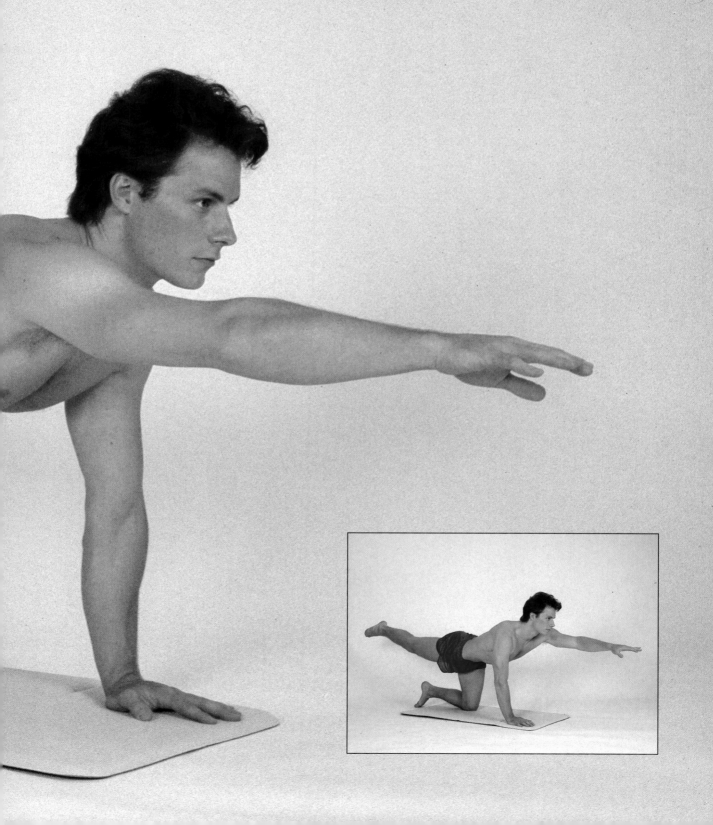

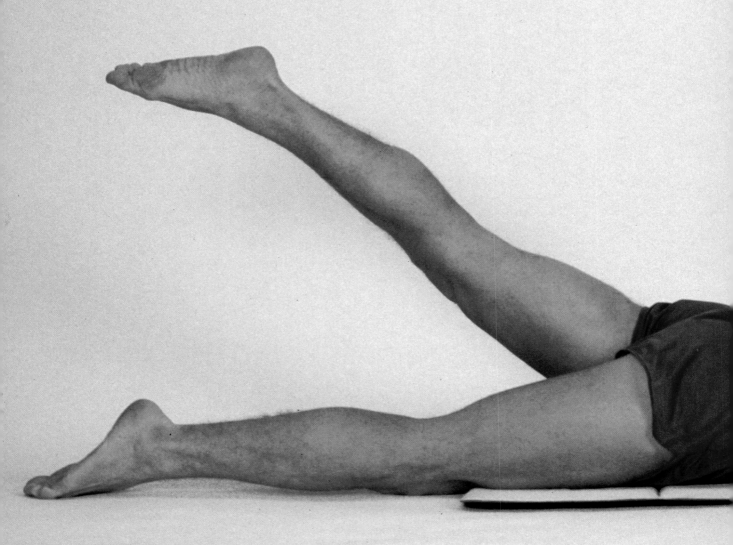

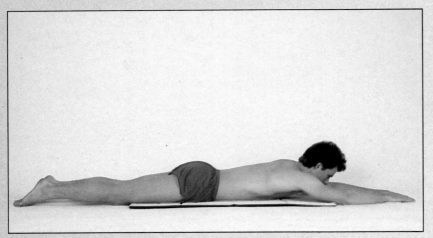

Diagonal Back Lift

Lie flat on your stomach with your hands stretched in front of your slightly lifted head *(left)*. Slowly raise your extended right arm and left leg, toes pointed, as high as possible without twisting your torso *(below)*. Lower and repeat with the other arm and leg *(inset opposite)*. Work up to three sets of 10 repetitions.

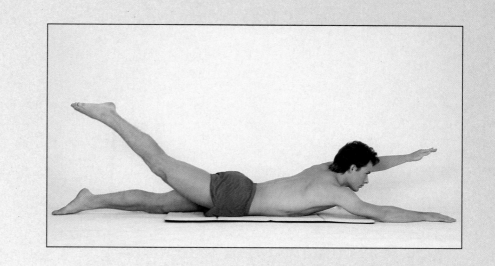

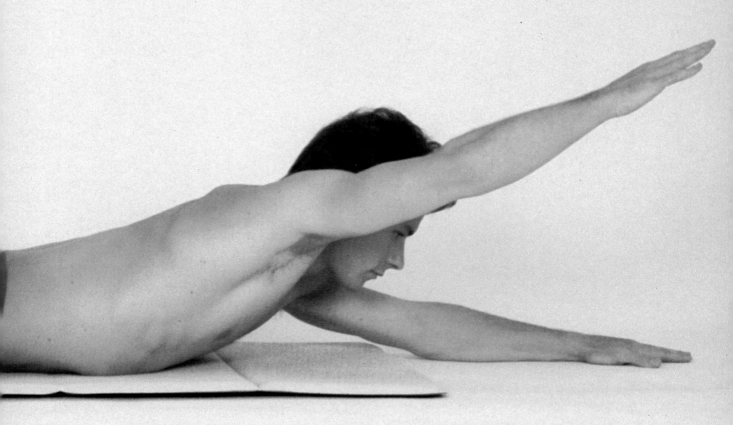

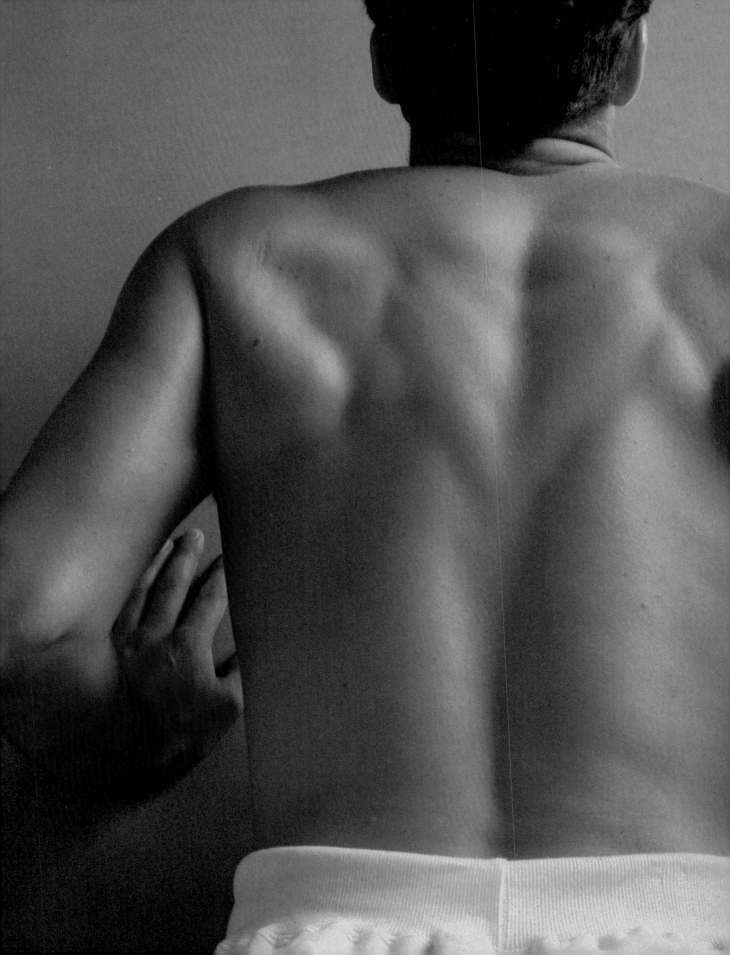

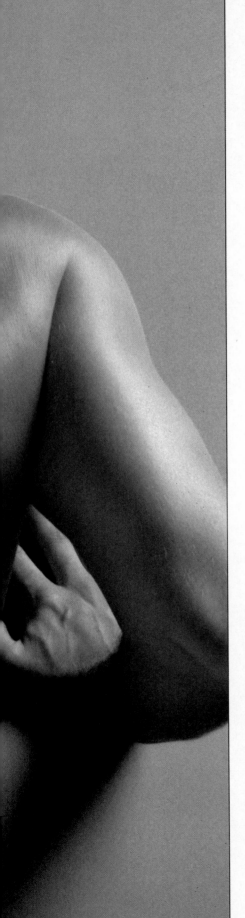

CHAPTER FOUR

The Upper Body

Broad shoulders, a taut chest and well-shaped arms — the right way

To most of us not well versed in anatomy, the biceps, triceps and pectorals are probably the best-known muscles in the body. They, along with the deltoids and trapezius of the shoulder and the latissimus of the back, are the muscles associated with a classic physique. Yet studies show that the upper body suffers the most neglect. People who make the effort to do something about their waistlines may be unable to do a single push-up. Women are especially weak in upper body strength, with slackness along the back of the upper arm a common problem. And men whose biceps are firm from regular use may have weak, shapeless muscles in their shoulders, chest and back.

Precisely because they are often the most neglected, the muscles in the upper body often respond most quickly to conditioning, and the results can be impressive. That this area generally stores less fat than other areas also makes the results of exercise appear more readily.

The illustration on page 97 shows how these muscles shape your upper body. At the back of your shoulders and neck, and descending between your shoulder blades, is the trapezius. It draws your head back, rotates your head and shrugs your shoulders. The deltoids shape the tops and sides of the shoulders. They lift your arms to the side, help raise them above your head, and swing them forward and back. The biceps, the familiar two-headed muscle in your upper arm, lifts your forearm. The three-part triceps, covering most of the back of your upper arm, opposes the biceps to straighten the arm.

Your chest and back are shaped by much larger muscles. The pectoralis major, the big muscle of your chest, moves your arms front and center and gives you force to push. (In birds, the pectorals are the muscles of flight, powering the wings.) The latissimus dorsi covers a broad portion of your back. Although activities like chopping wood or swinging a pickax work this muscle, it is generally underexercised, and its weakness often contributes to shoulder problems. The teres major and the rhomboids, which act on the shoulder blade, also frequently suffer from disuse and from being forced into the hunched-over position associated with sitting at a desk all day.

Exercising these muscles produces notable improvements in appearance as well as strength. Developing the latissimus dorsi, for example, gives definition to your middle back and strengthens your pulling power. It is the latissimus that produces a classic V-shaped torso, which you can accentuate with broader-looking shoulders by working the deltoids. Firmer backs of upper arms are another benefit: Because the triceps, the muscle that shapes that area, generally gets little work from day-to-day routines, it frequently responds quickly to toning.

A toned chest, a result of working the pectorals, improves the appearance of both sexes. Women may notice that pectoral exercises make their breasts look firmer and higher as they receive better support from underlying tissue. Improving the tone of upper body muscles will also enhance your posture. Toned muscles hold your head more erect, lift your upper chest and draw your shoulders down and back. And people of both sexes will find that any number of daily tasks, from carrying groceries to opening heavy doors, become easier.

Women worry needlessly that they will become overdeveloped from working their upper bodies. For muscle to bulk up heavily, high levels of testosterone, a male sex hormone, are required. (Women's bodies do produce testosterone, but in minute quantities.) Men who do not wish to look like power lifters can also relax: The exercises in this chapter do not lead to excessive muscle growth.

Because people differ in their strength and their goals, this chapter contains a wide range of exercises. In addition to helping you avoid the tedium of performing the same routine, variety is necessary for dealing with the complexity of the upper body. Many people will choose to start their routines with the push-up (*pages 100-107*). This versatile exercise, which requires little or no equipment, combines work for shoulders, chest and arms, and has variations that may be used to emphasize the triceps, deltoids or pectorals. In addition, ab-

Upper Body

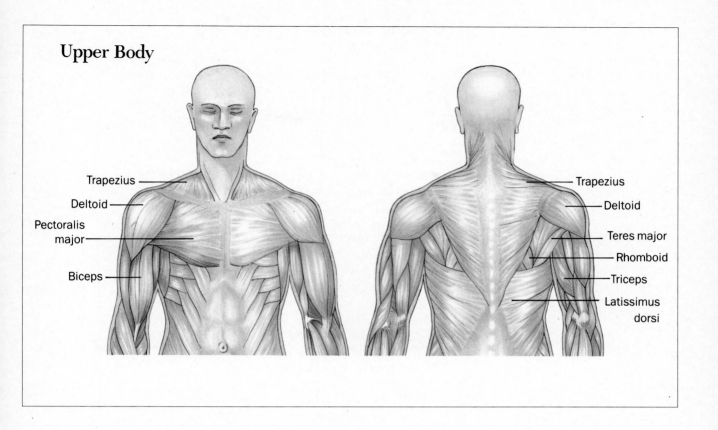

Trapezius
Deltoid
Pectoralis major
Biceps

Trapezius
Deltoid
Teres major
Rhomboid
Triceps
Latissimus dorsi

dominal muscles, gluteals and leg extensors must work hard to hold your body rigid for the push-up.

You should pair any pushing exercise with a pulling exercise to prevent imbalances that put weaker muscles in jeopardy. Good exercises to oppose the push-up are the dip *(pages 108-109)* or the chin-up, which may also be done as a bent-arm hang *(pages 122-123)*. Both strengthen a weak latissimus. In addition, the chin-up works the major flexors of the arm, including the biceps, while the dip works the triceps harder. You can also do pulling work with weights in a bent-over position *(pages 112-113)*.

In upper body work, you may exercise either the latissimus or the pectorals of the chest first, since both are large muscles. Bench presses and bench flys *(pages 110-111)* target the pectorals if you want to intensify or concentrate on chest work. The lift to the front with the weight bar (which may also be performed with dumbbells) is a good choice for combining chest and shoulder work *(page 120)*.

It is particularly important in working this part of the body to maintain your position as you perform the exercises. Leaning forward and backward when doing curls, for instance, not only makes the exercise easier and hence less effective by dividing the work among a number of bigger muscles, but it may also cause back strain. And if you cheat by not performing exercises through the full range of motion, you may shorten your muscles and deprive yourself of flexibility.

Warm-Ups

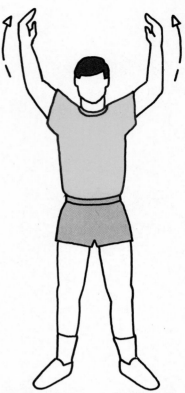

Because arms and shoulders are often the least-exercised body areas, they are the most likely to suffer stiffness and injury if you do not warm them up properly. Poor posture and day-to-day muscular tension also particularly afflict the upper body. In fact, quite a few muscular athletes are stiff in this area because they fail to stretch it properly.

You can prevent trouble by performing the movements shown on these two pages. As an added bonus, this routine will help increase your lung capacity.

Before you start, jog in place, swinging your arms vigorously to get blood flowing to upper body muscles and to limber upper body joints.

When you are finished, repeat the stretching sequence of the last three movements. Muscles that have just been worked will stretch with greater ease.

Swing your arms from above your head to across your chest *(above and right)*. **Keep the flow of motion smooth — do not stop moving. Perform 30 repetitions.**

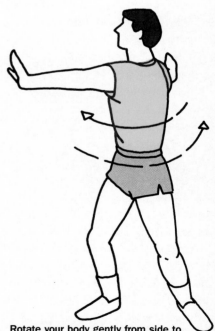

Rotate your body gently from side to side 30 times *(above)*. **Deepen the bend of your knees at the end of each twist.**

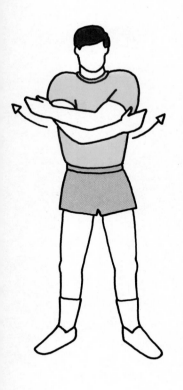

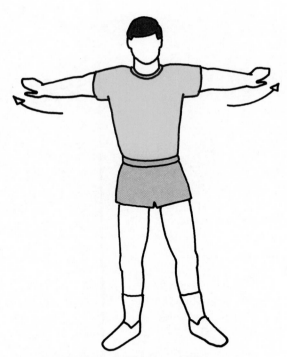

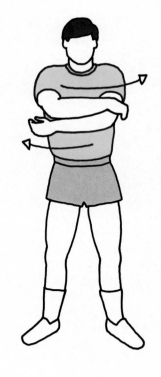

Swing your arms back and forth 30 times *(above and right)*. Swing at a moderate pace. Do not strain to reach back or fling your arms with excessive force.

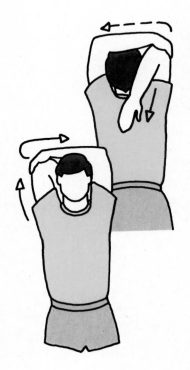

To help stretch shoulder joints, reach down the middle of your back with your right hand *(left)*. With your left arm, reach over your head and pull your elbow gently to the left for 20 seconds. Repeat the stretch on the other side.

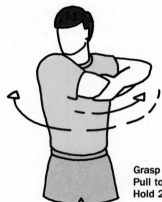

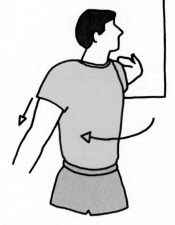

With your left hand on a wall, turn your torso to the right *(above)*. Pull your right shoulder back and down. Reverse hands.

Grasp your arms above your elbows *(left)*. Pull to the left, turning your head right. Hold 20 seconds, then pull to the right.

The Push-Up

Push-ups can quickly strengthen shoulders, arms and chest. Using the weight of your body for resistance, this classic exercise overloads the front deltoids, pectorals and triceps. Tiring these muscles fast makes them respond rapidly if they are out of shape. Moreover, push-ups work abdominal and back muscles, which stabilize your body and keep it rigid during the exercise. Even your legs and buttocks get a workout.

In addition to quick, effective strengthening, adaptability is one of the push-up's advantages. No matter how strong or weak you are, one of the variations here and on the following six pages will help tone you. And by shifting to different positions, you can use push-ups to concentrate the work on your deltoids, pectorals or triceps.

The push-up is not an easy exercise. Many women cannot initially do one full push-up, and men who do not exercise their upper bodies regularly may also have trouble. But after having practiced the modified push-up here until you can do 20 without pause, you should be able to master the classic push-up *(pages 102-103)*. If even the modified version is too taxing, do the exercise while standing up and leaning against a wall. Increase the angle and the number of repetitions until you can switch to the floor. Later you can vary the push-up to increase its intensity or to focus on muscles you want to target.

Do the modified push-up on your knees with your hands underneath your shoulders and your ankles crossed. Keep your torso straight as you lower your chest to the floor *(inset)* and push back up. Do not lock your elbows in the up position *(right)*.

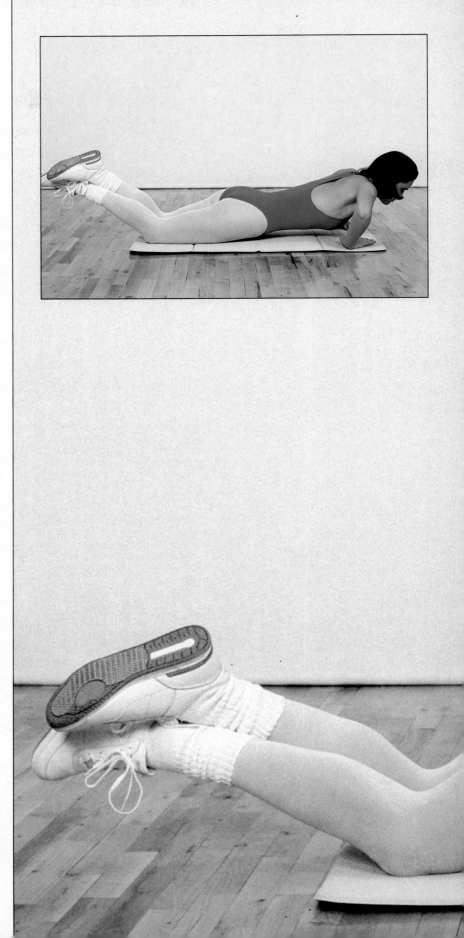

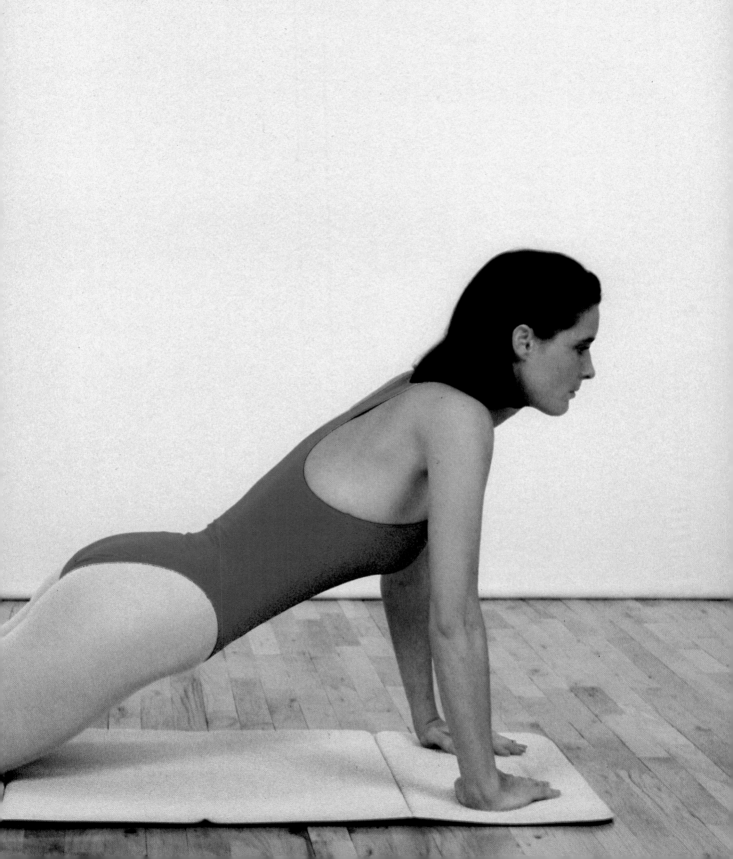

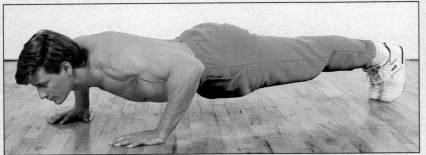

The Classic Push-Up

To concentrate work on the front of your shoulders, balance your weight between your hands (placed under shoulders) and your toes, which are flexed. Align your body so that it is straight *(below)*. Keep it rigid as you lower your chest to the floor *(left)*. Do not rest between push-ups or lock your elbows.

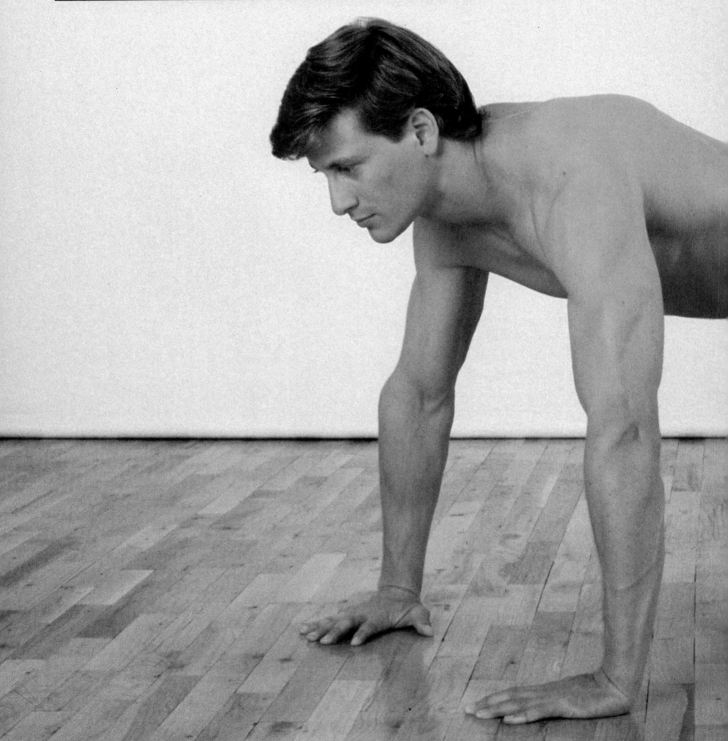

To work on your chest, space your
hands widely, point your fingers straight
ahead and hold your elbows close to
your body *(top right)*. A close-grip
push-up shapes and tones triceps faster
(bottom right).

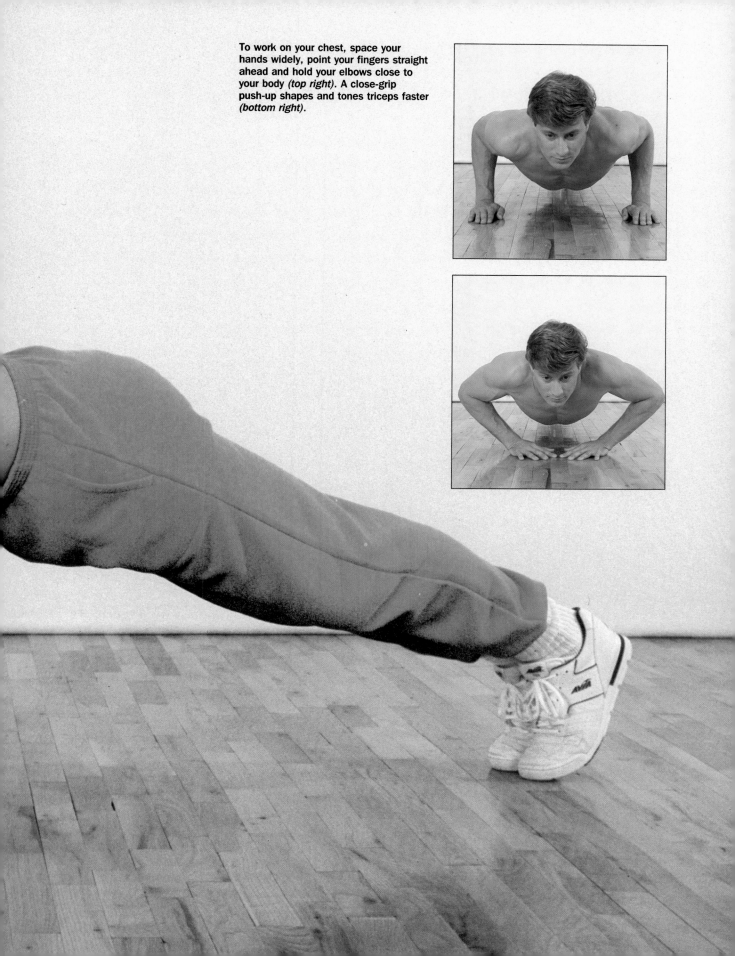

The Deltoid Push-Up

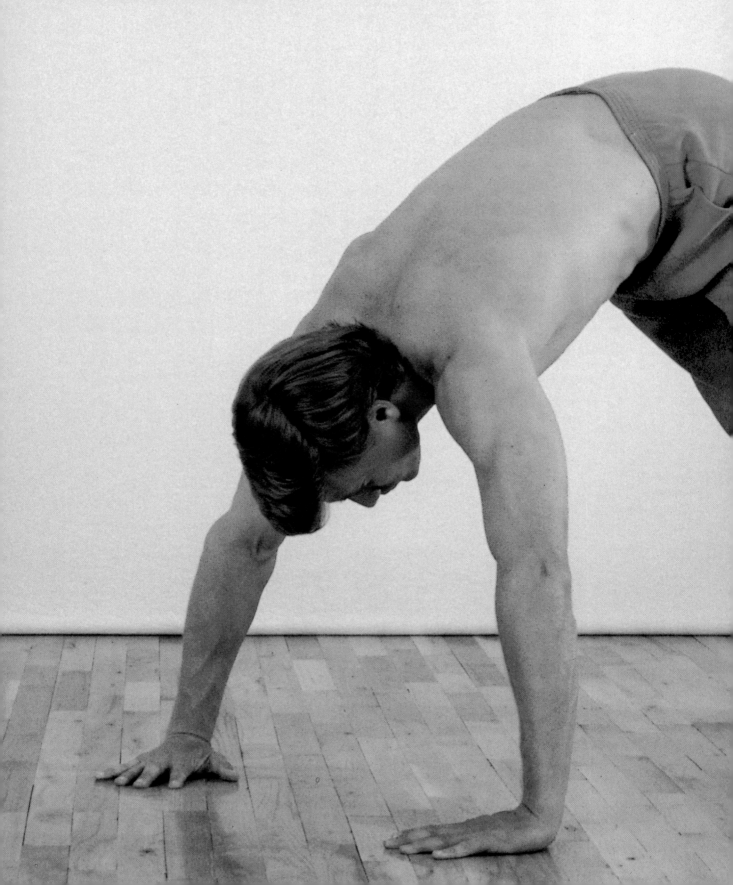

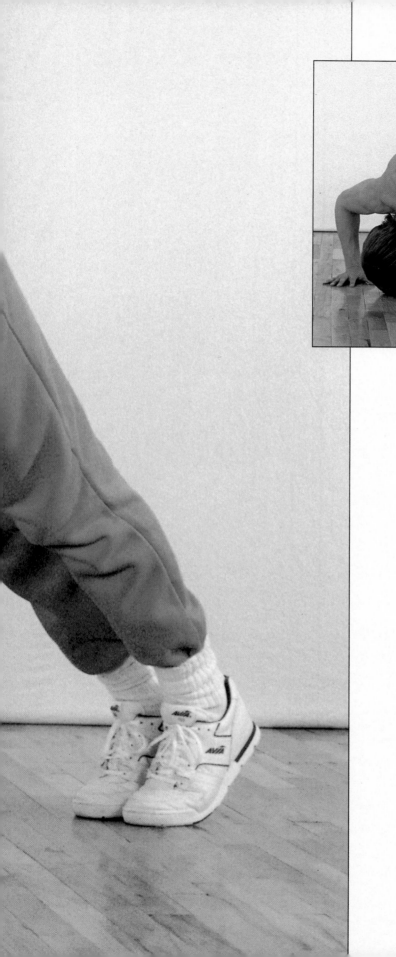

By bringing the weight of your torso to bear on your shoulders, this push-up tones the deltoids and also firms the trapezius. Make your body into a bridge, bending at the hip and dividing your weight between your hands and toes. Keep your elbows slightly bent even when you are fully raised *(left)*. Keep your body bent at the same angle as you slowly lower yourself toward the floor *(above)*.

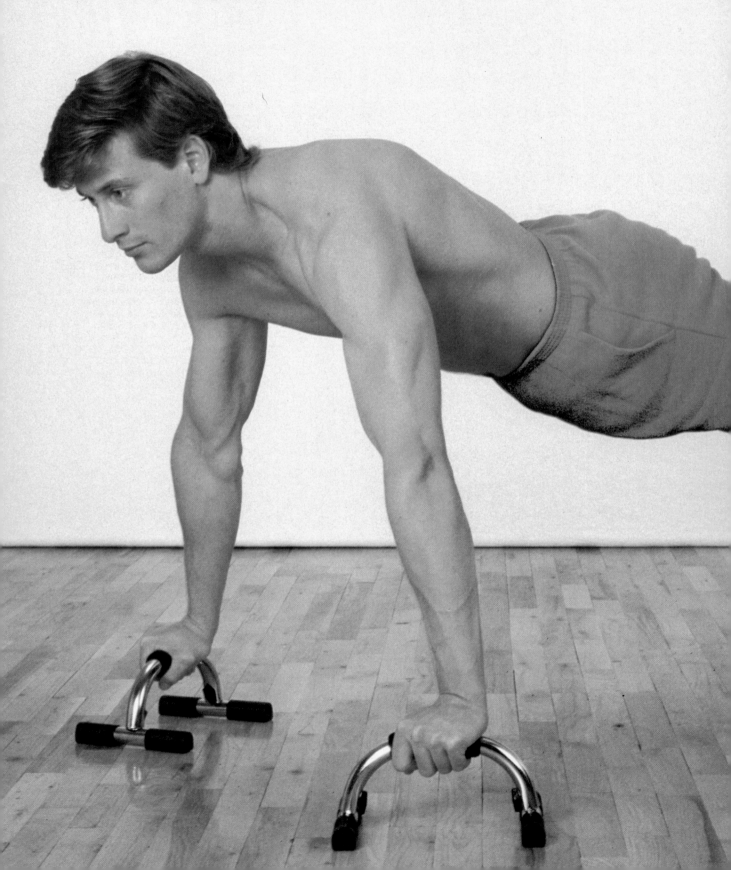

The Raised Push-Up

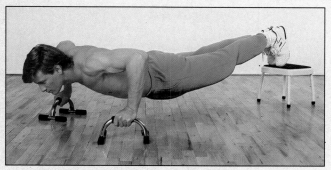

Place arm lifters at a right angle to each other and spaced slightly wider than your shoulders *(below)*. Lower yourself as far as you can without bending your body *(above)*.

When doing push-ups with your feet lifted, maintain rigidity in your back as you lift and lower *(below and bottom)*, but do not hyperextend your elbows. The higher you raise your feet, the more weight shifts onto your upper body, intensifying the effort. Similarly, by allowing you to descend lower, lifters — or any sturdy, untippable hand supports — intensify work for your arms, back and chest. The ultimate upper body builder is a handstand push-up done against a wall. But most people will find the versions shown here sufficiently challenging.

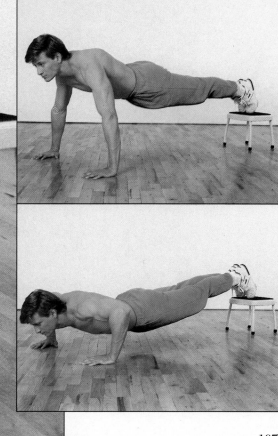

The Dip

An extremely effective exercise that requires no equipment, the dip focuses effort on the rear deltoids, lower pectorals, triceps, lower trapezius and latissimus — important shapers of the shoulders, arms, chest and back. Like the push-up, the dip uses body weight to overload muscles that do not usually have to provide much support. When performing the dip, use a weight bench, a stool or a sturdy, well-balanced chair.

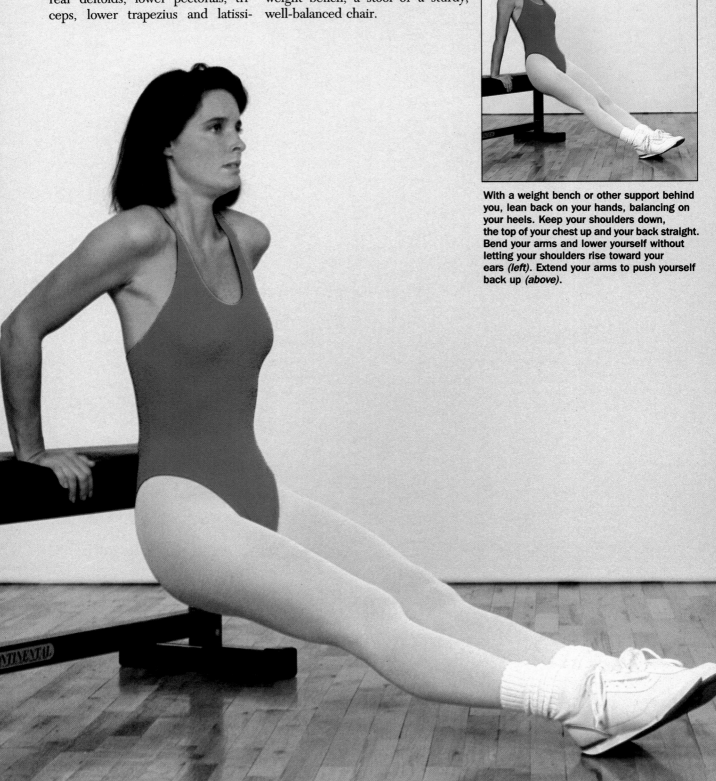

With a weight bench or other support behind you, lean back on your hands, balancing on your heels. Keep your shoulders down, the top of your chest up and your back straight. Bend your arms and lower yourself without letting your shoulders rise toward your ears *(left)*. Extend your arms to push yourself back up *(above)*.

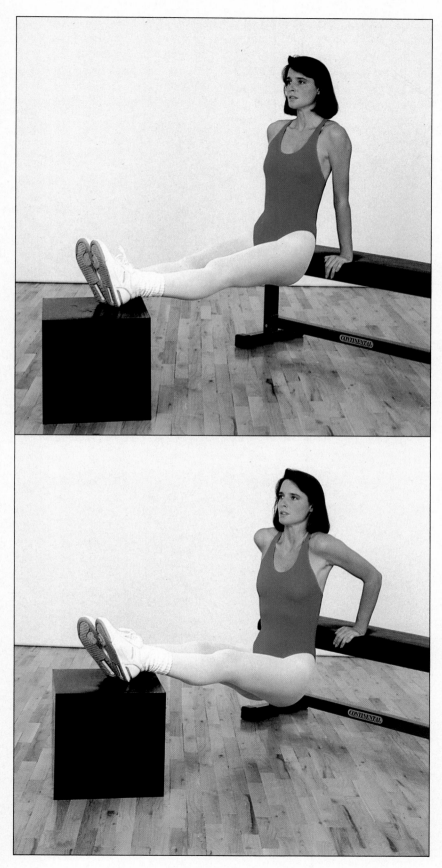

Elevating your feet for dips adds lower body weight to the exercise, making it harder. Lean on your hands and place your heels on the support *(top left)*. Dip without allowing your shoulders to rise *(bottom left)*, then push back up.

Small Weights

Using small weights lets you work isolated muscles better than exercises that rely on body weight alone. You can, for instance, isolate the triceps to firm the back of your arms. Concentration curls target your biceps. Three- to five-pound weights work well for most women, though many will want heavier loads for bench and military presses and for upright and bent-over rows. Most men will prefer seven- to 10-pound dumbbells for flys, curls and single weight lifts, but may want to use heavier weights in the same exercises as women.

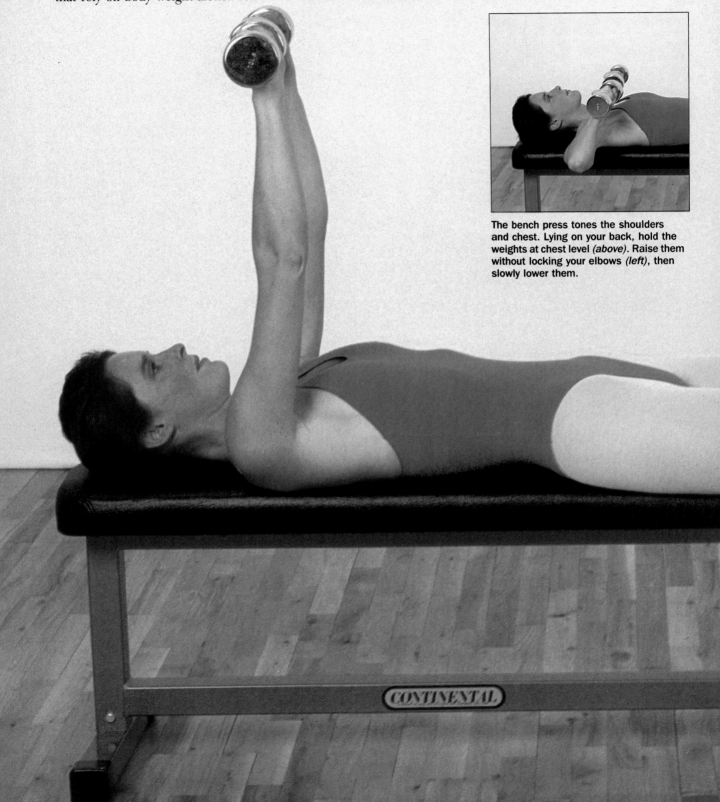

The bench press tones the shoulders and chest. Lying on your back, hold the weights at chest level *(above)*. Raise them without locking your elbows *(left)*, then slowly lower them.

Bench flys isolate the pectorals, the major muscles that shape the chest. Hold your arms out to your sides, forming a cross *(top left)*. Keep your elbows slightly bent and your back flat on the bench. Lift the weights through a semicircular arch until they are side by side above your chest *(top right)*. Breathe evenly throughout the work. To isolate your triceps, grasp both ends of a single dumbbell high over your chest *(middle right)*. Keep your upper arms still and lower the weight several inches behind your head with your forearms until they form a right angle *(middle left)*. To exercise your latissimus, thereby shaping your back and sides, hold one end of a dumbbell in both hands as far as you can to the rear of your head *(bottom left)*. Slowly raise the dumbbell until it is over your chest *(bottom right)*. Keep your elbows unlocked.

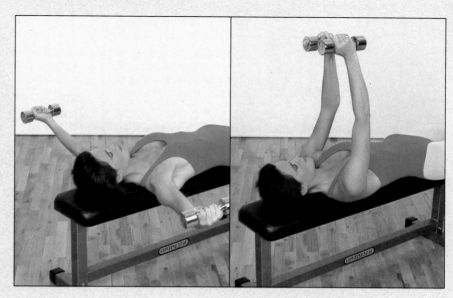

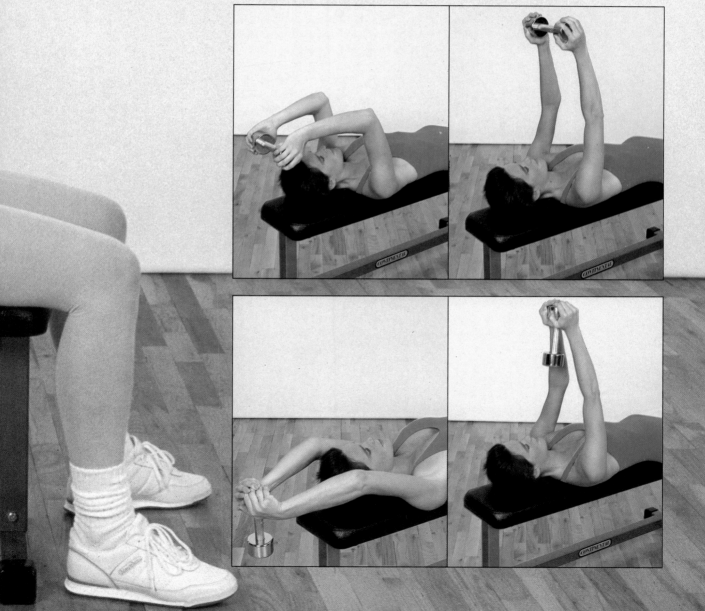

Bent-Over Lifts

To do a bent-over row, which will firm your latissimus, trapezius, rhomboid and biceps, bend your knees and lean forward at the hip. Keep your back straight and buttocks high. Let the weights hang down, but keep your elbows slightly bent *(left)*. Lift weights straight up *(below)*.

Single rows *(below and bottom)* stabilize your body, focus the effort on one side and protect the lower back. Bend over with your knee and hand on a weight bench.

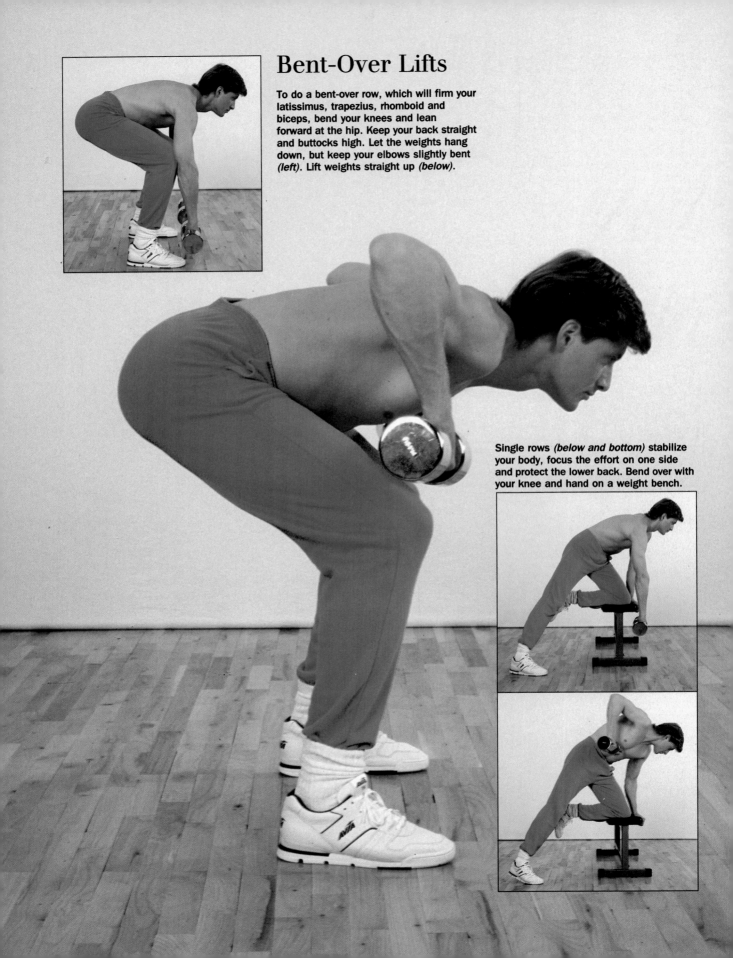

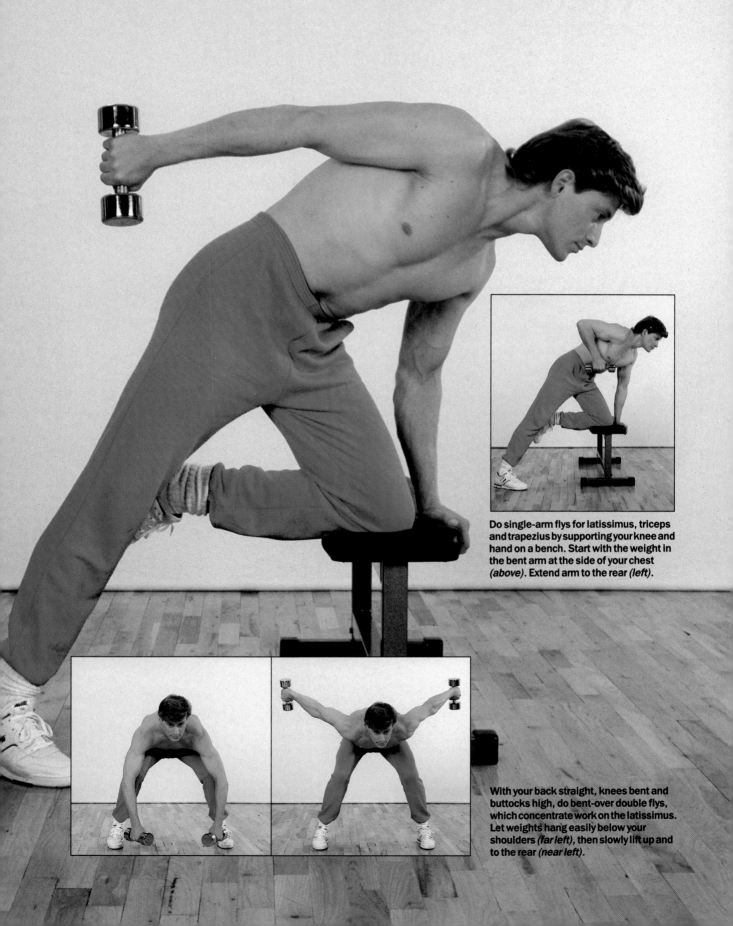

Do single-arm flys for latissimus, triceps and trapezius by supporting your knee and hand on a bench. Start with the weight in the bent arm at the side of your chest *(above)*. Extend arm to the rear *(left)*.

With your back straight, knees bent and buttocks high, do bent-over double flys, which concentrate work on the latissimus. Let weights hang easily below your shoulders *(far left)*, then slowly lift up and to the rear *(near left)*.

Standing Lifts

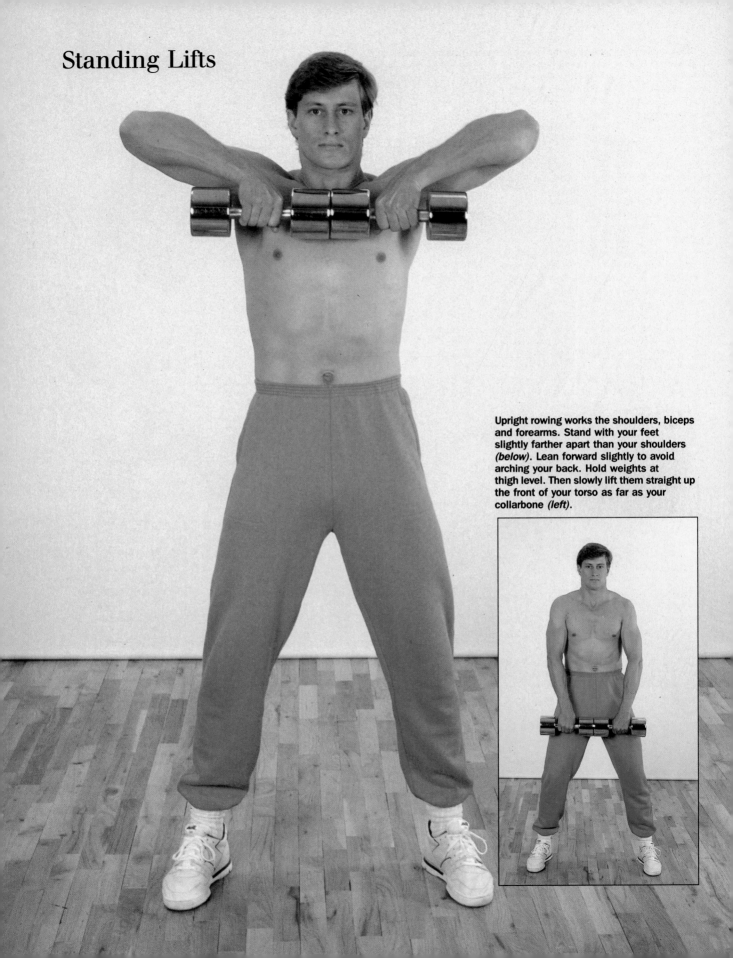

Upright rowing works the shoulders, biceps and forearms. Stand with your feet slightly farther apart than your shoulders *(below)*. Lean forward slightly to avoid arching your back. Hold weights at thigh level. Then slowly lift them straight up the front of your torso as far as your collarbone *(left)*.

To do a lateral raise, stand with the same relaxed good posture as described opposite, but with dumbbells parallel to each other *(below left)*. **Slowly lift out to the sides to focus work on the deltoids** *(below right)*. **Keep your elbows slightly bent.**

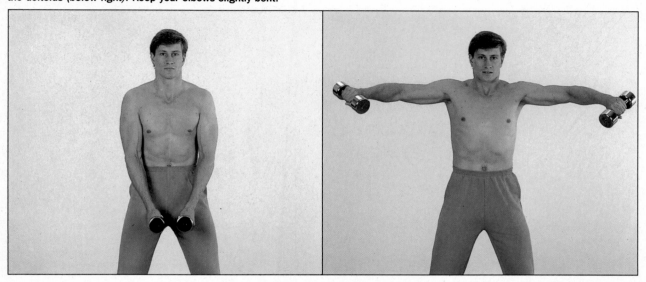

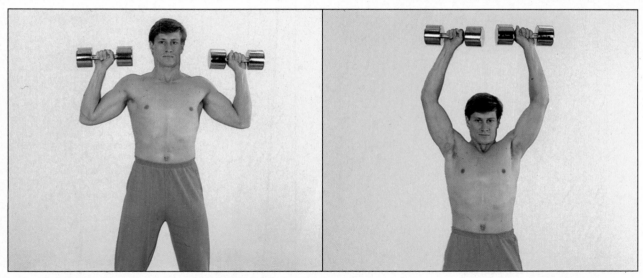

For the military press, hold the dumbbells horizontally a few inches above your shoulder *(above left)*. Slowly raise them straight up without locking your elbows or arching your lower back *(above right)*.

Biceps and Triceps Lifts

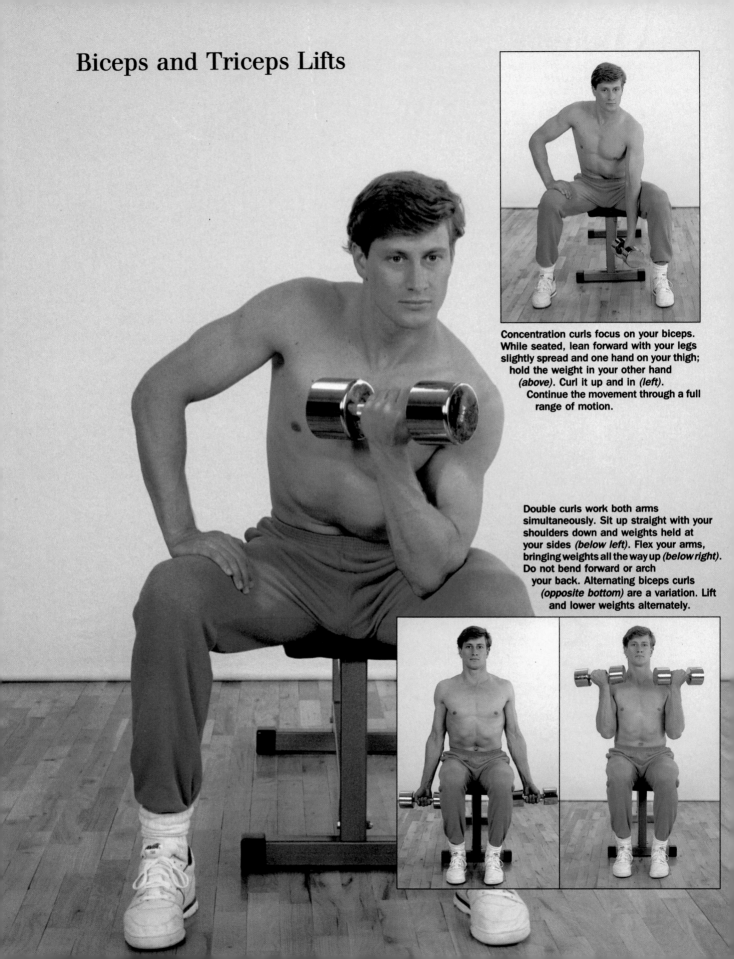

Concentration curls focus on your biceps. While seated, lean forward with your legs slightly spread and one hand on your thigh; hold the weight in your other hand *(above)*. Curl it up and in *(left)*. Continue the movement through a full range of motion.

Double curls work both arms simultaneously. Sit up straight with your shoulders down and weights held at your sides *(below left)*. Flex your arms, bringing weights all the way up *(below right)*. Do not bend forward or arch your back. Alternating biceps curls *(opposite bottom)* are a variation. Lift and lower weights alternately.

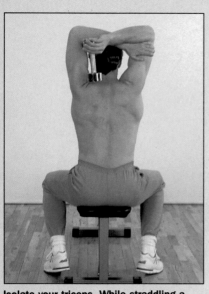

Isolate your triceps. While straddling a bench with your back straight, fold your arms over your head. Hold the end of the dumbbell in one hand and use the other hand to steady the weight-bearing arm *(above)*. Raise your arm without locking your elbow *(right)*.

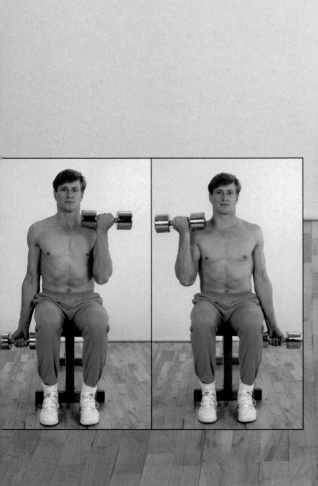

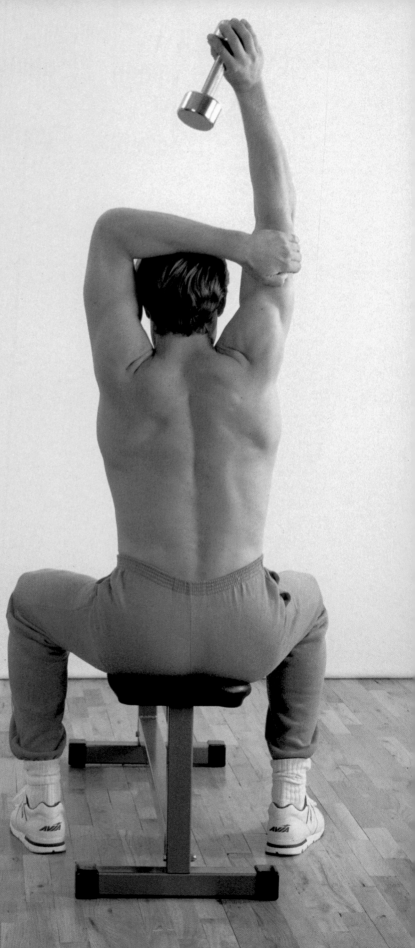

Bar Lifts/1

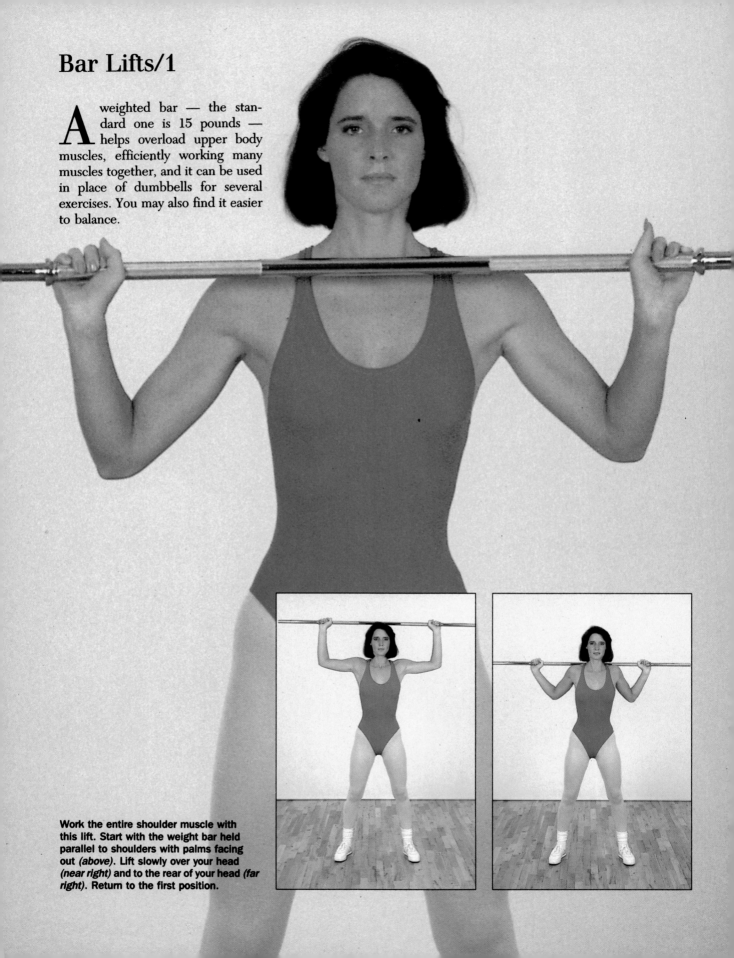

A weighted bar — the standard one is 15 pounds — helps overload upper body muscles, efficiently working many muscles together, and it can be used in place of dumbbells for several exercises. You may also find it easier to balance.

Work the entire shoulder muscle with this lift. Start with the weight bar held parallel to shoulders with palms facing out *(above)*. Lift slowly over your head *(near right)* and to the rear of your head *(far right)*. Return to the first position.

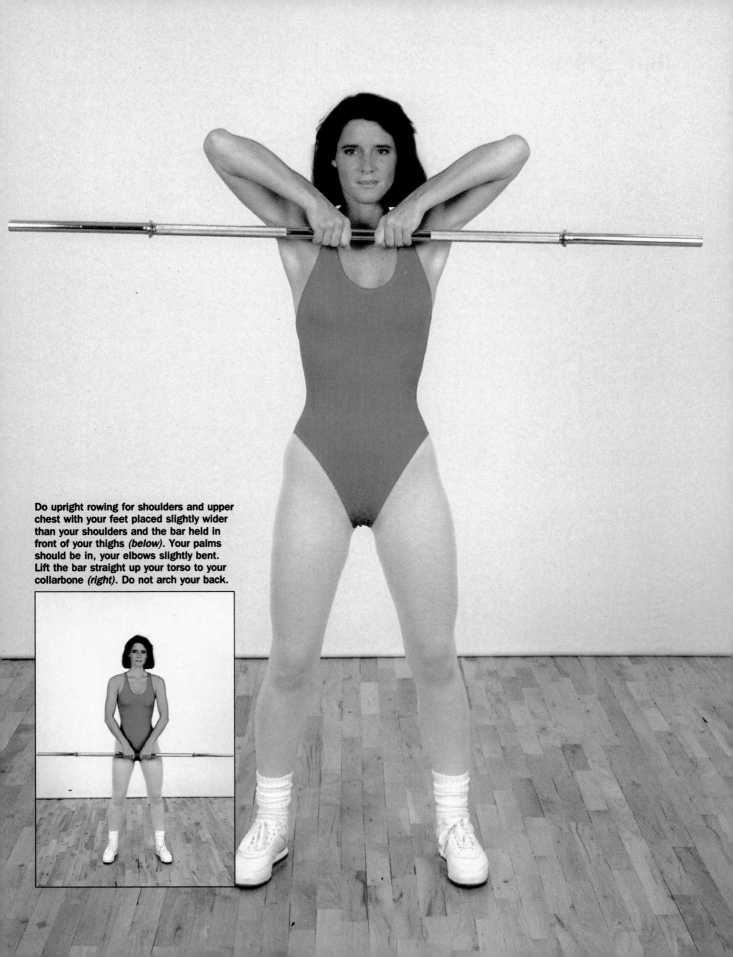

Do upright rowing for shoulders and upper chest with your feet placed slightly wider than your shoulders and the bar held in front of your thighs *(below)*. Your palms should be in, your elbows slightly bent. Lift the bar straight up your torso to your collarbone *(right)*. Do not arch your back.

Bar Lifts/2

Work front deltoids and upper pectorals with a forward lift while seated. Hold the bar at neck level with palms facing forward *(below left)*. Extend your arms out and up so the bar is slightly above your head *(below right)*.

Do a behind-the-head press to focus on rear deltoids and trapezius. Start with the bar at neck level and your hands spaced far apart *(bottom left)*; lift straight up *(bottom right)*. Be sure that you do not lock your elbows.

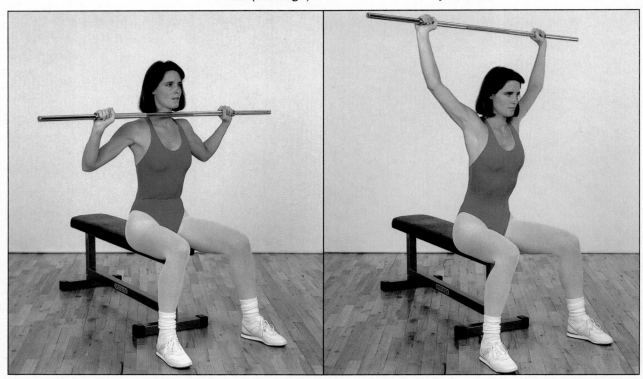

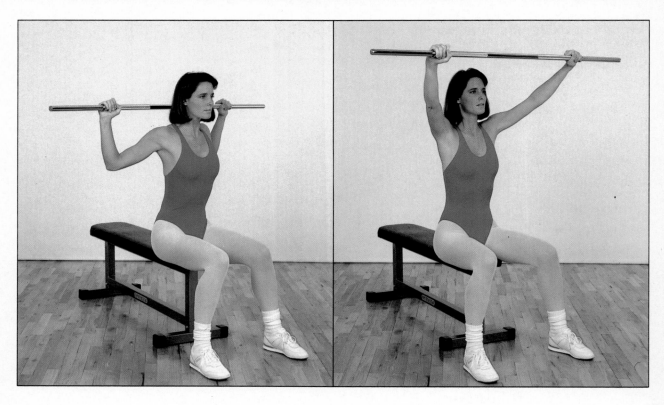

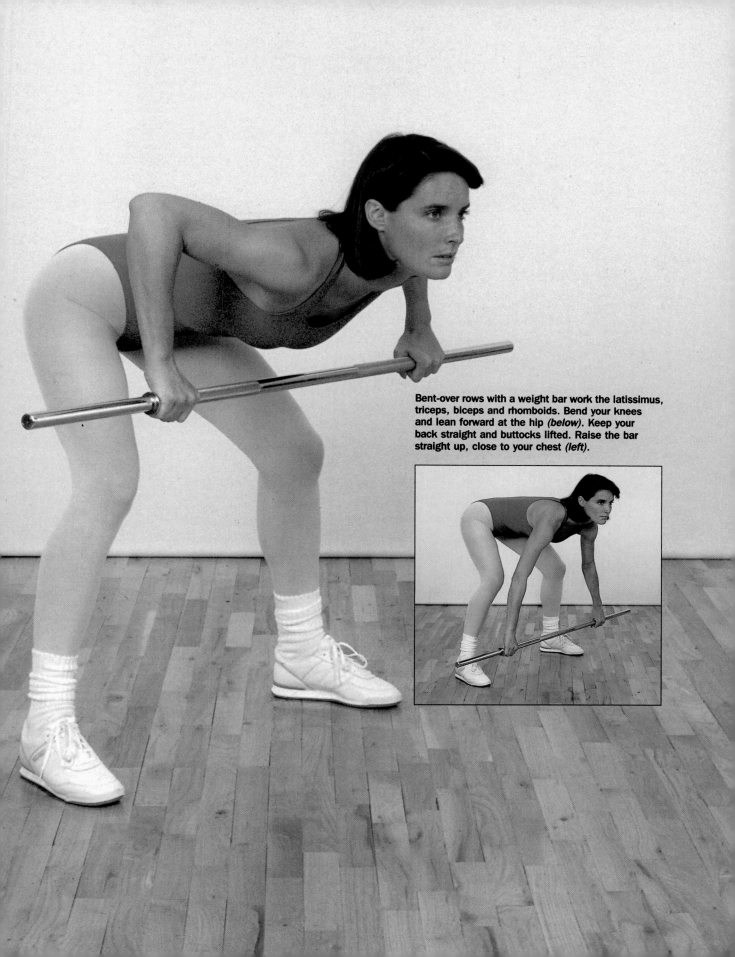

Bent-over rows with a weight bar work the latissimus, triceps, biceps and rhomboids. Bend your knees and lean forward at the hip *(below)*. Keep your back straight and buttocks lifted. Raise the bar straight up, close to your chest *(left)*.

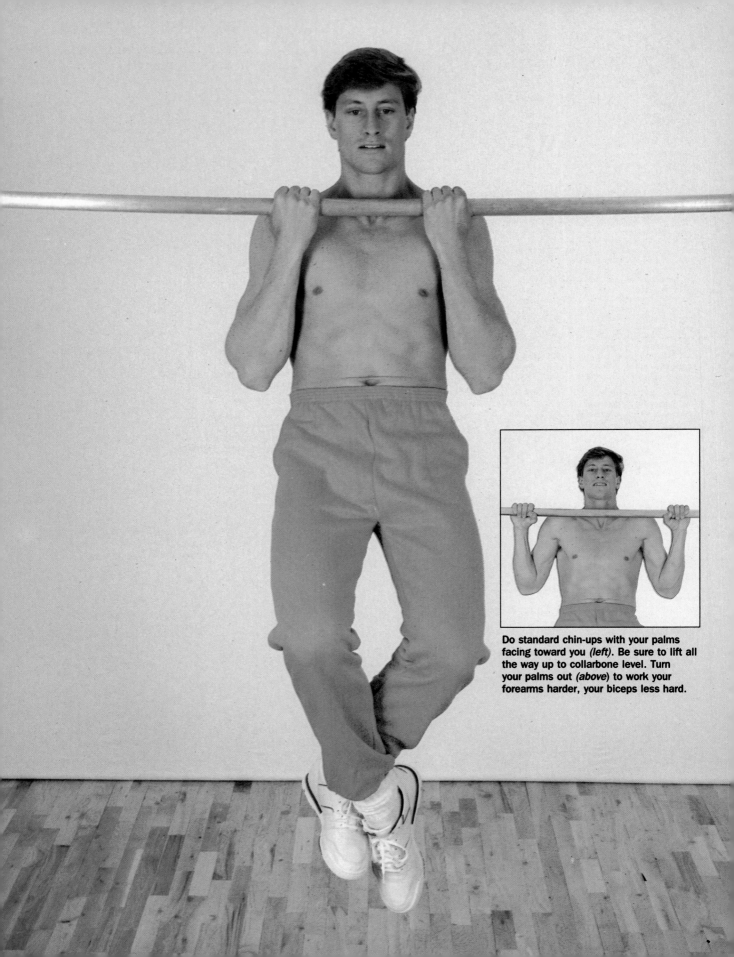

Do standard chin-ups with your palms facing toward you *(left)*. Be sure to lift all the way up to collarbone level. Turn your palms out *(above)* to work your forearms harder, your biceps less hard.

Chinning

With a chinning bar, you can use your entire weight for upper body resistance. The chin-up quickly gives muscles an intense workout. A chin-up requires so much strength, however, that most women and some men will have to work up to it. But even the easiest version, the supported bent-arm hang, can give you a good workout, and you can stay with it if you find it sufficiently intense. (To increase strength and tone, you can extend the time you hang.)

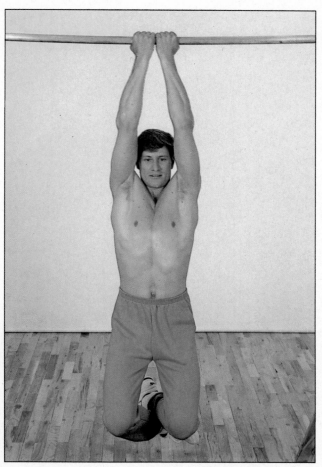

A bent-arm hang with your legs supported is the easiest way to work the chinning bar. Place your feet or calves on a stable object to support part of your weight *(below)*. Hold the bar with palms in, elbows bent. Hang in this position for 30 seconds or as long as you comfortably can. Rest 30 seconds and repeat. When you can do this easily, chin yourself with your legs supported.

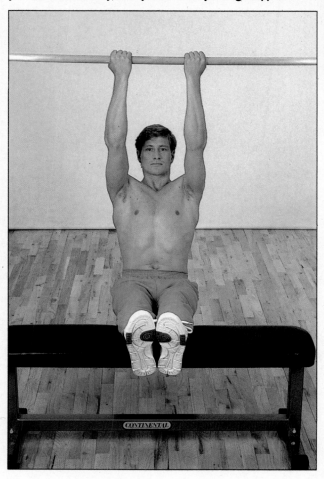

A bent-arm hang with legs free is the next level of difficulty. Grasp the bar with your palms facing in and your elbows bent slightly. Lift your legs and hang for as long as you can *(above)*. Work up to 45 seconds; when you can hang for that long, try a full chin-up.

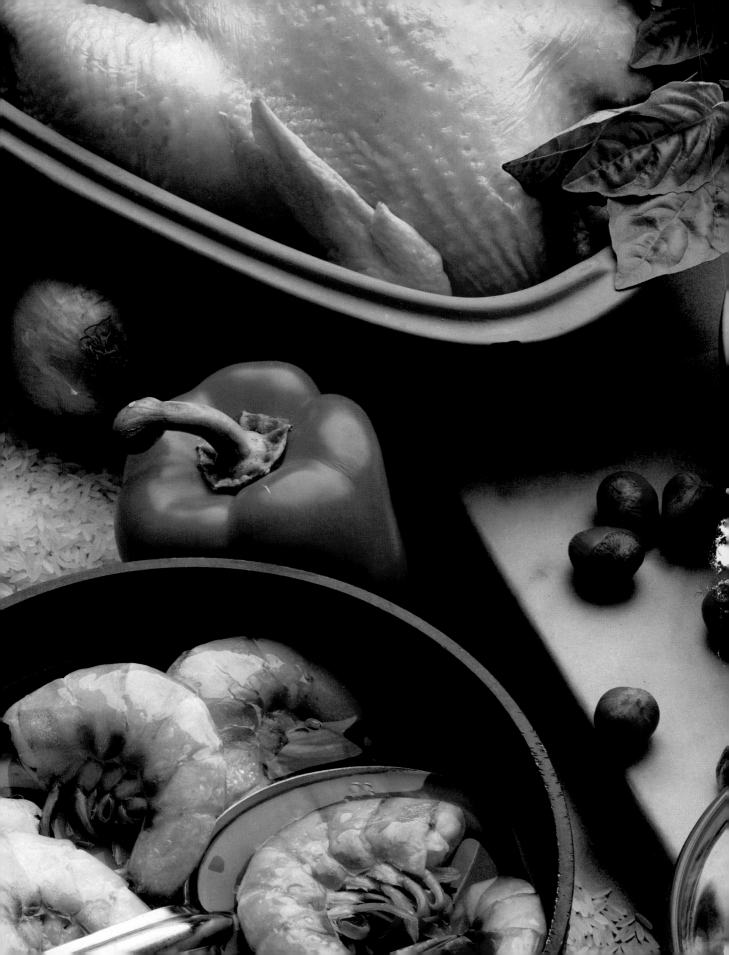

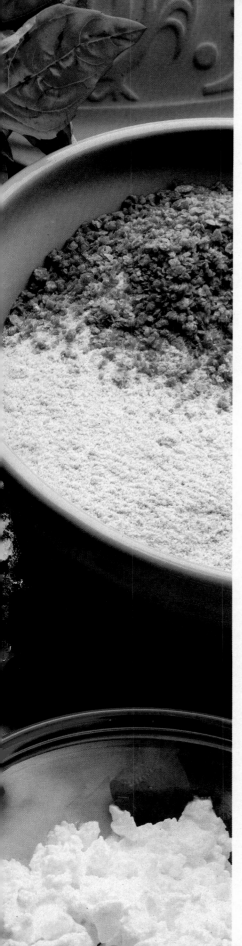

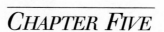

CHAPTER FIVE

Protein

The essential — but often overused — nutrient for muscle

P rotein is the basic building block of the human body. It forms the substance of our muscles, organs, antibodies and enzymes (the compounds that control our interior chemical reactions). As these structures break down and are repaired, most of their protein is recycled and used again. But we cannot store protein, so the lost material, the protein "turnover," has to be constantly replaced by protein digested from our food. While foods derived from meat have the highest proportion of protein, foods derived from plants can also supply a more than adequate amount.

Certain parts of our body, such as muscles, use more protein than others. The large muscles that weight lifters and body builders develop represent large bundles of added protein. In addition to forming tissue, protein acts as a source of energy for exercise, although its role is secondary to that of carbohydrates and fats.

Since muscles are made of protein, athletes in search of extra strength and muscle size sometimes consume two to three times the

The following foods are all high in protein and low in cholesterol and saturated fat.

DAIRY PRODUCTS:

Skim milk
Lowfat yogurt

FISH:

Tuna
Flounder

POULTRY:

Turkey
Chicken

VEGETARIAN FOODS:

Brown rice
Buckwheat
High-protein pasta
Oats
Soybean sprouts
Tofu

recommended amount of protein. But eating a lot of protein does not improve power or endurance. The only way to make a particular muscle bigger is to exercise it. Consuming a lot of protein-rich foods only causes the body to manufacture new layers of fat.

When we eat protein, we do not absorb it directly. Our digestive system first separates it into amino acids — the components of all proteins. After digestion, the body recombines these acids into the particular protein compounds it needs. Although amino acids are fairly simple structures, they join in an almost infinite variety of long, often-complicated chains to create thousands of different proteins.

Of the 22 amino acids that scientists have identified, the human body can manufacture 13. The other nine acids, the so-called essential amino acids, cannot be made; the diet must supply them. Foods or meals that contain all nine essential amino acids are said to provide "complete" protein. Your body can use the amino acids in these foods to make any protein it requires. "Incomplete" protein lacks one or more of the essential amino acids. And without these, the body cannot piece together all the proteins it needs for good health.

All red meat contains complete protein; so do other animal products, such as fish, milk, eggs and poultry. Almost no single plant food, except for some legumes, does. To get the best use of the protein from vegetables and grains, you have to eat them with animal foods or in complementary combinations that include the nine essential amino acids. Designing meatless, vegetarian meals and dishes that meet this requirement is not difficult. The general rule is to eat a serving of legumes, such as beans, lentils, peanuts or peas, with a helping of corn or a grain, such as rice or wheat. By themselves, most legumes and grains are incomplete proteins. When properly combined, they supply all the essential amino acids, and common vegetarian dishes from almost every region of the world follow this dietary strategy.

While most of the protein-source calories in a healthy diet should come from vegetarian foods, your meals should also include a moderate amount of meat, eggs, milk, poultry and fish. Eating complete animal protein during mostly vegetarian meals helps your body make better use of the amino acids in plant foods. For instance, drinking a small amount of milk with potatoes enables your body to use the incomplete protein in potatoes more efficiently. You can eliminate a great deal of the harmful fat and cholesterol from animal foods by sticking to cuts of lean meat, eating three eggs or fewer per week, using skim milk products and eating more fish and poultry than red meat.

Moderate exercise increases your need for protein, but most people eat more than enough to compensate for this extra demand. The average person requires slightly more than a third of a gram of protein per pound of body weight every day. Dividing your weight by three gives you your approximate daily requirement in grams. A 150-pound man should have 50 to 60 grams a day; a 120-pound woman, 40 to 50 grams. Two to three servings of animal products or four servings of vegetarian foods easily fulfill the protein requirement of most adults.

The Basic Guidelines

For a moderately active adult, the National Institutes of Health recommends a diet that is low in fat, high in carbohydrates and moderate in protein. The institutes' guidelines suggest that no more than 30 percent of your calories come from fat, that 55 percent to 60 percent come from carbohydrates and that no more than 15 percent come from protein. A gram of fat equals nine calories, while a gram of protein or carbohydrate equals four calories; therefore, if you eat 2,100 calories a day, you should consume approximately 60 grams of fat, 315 grams of carbohydrate and no more than 75 grams of protein daily. If you follow a lowfat/high-carbohydrate diet, your chance of developing heart disease, cancer and other life-threatening diseases may be considerably reduced.

The nutrition charts that accompany each of the lowfat/high-carbohydrate recipes in this book include the number of calories per serving, the number of grams of fat, carbohydrate and protein in a serving, and the percentage of calories derived from each of these nutrients. In addition, the charts provide the amount of calcium, iron and sodium per serving.

Calcium deficiency may be associated with periodontal disease — which attacks the mouth's bones and tissues, including the gums — in both men and women, and with osteoporosis, or bone shrinking and weakening, in the elderly. The deficiency may also contribute to high blood pressure. The recommended daily allowance for calcium is 800 milligrams a day for men and women. Pregnant and lactating women are advised to consume 1,200 milligrams daily; a National Institutes of Health consensus panel recommends that postmenopausal women consume 1,200 to 1,500 milligrams of calcium each day.

Although one way you can reduce your fat intake is to cut your consumption of red meat, you should make sure that you get your necessary iron from other sources. The Food and Nutrition Board of the National Academy of Sciences suggests a minimum of 10 milligrams of iron per day for men and 18 milligrams for women between the ages of 11 and 50.

High sodium intake is associated with high blood pressure. Most adults should restrict sodium intake to between 2,000 and 2,500 milligrams a day, according to the National Academy of Sciences. One way to keep sodium consumption in check is not to add table salt to food.

"Protein loading" does not grow bigger muscles or have any other useful function. And it can be dangerous. Besides being fattening, protein is toxic in large doses.

As long as you eat a balanced diet, it is the amount of carbohydrates you consume that allows protein to build muscle. While protein does play an important role in fueling exercise, adequate dietary carbohydrates enable the body to burn primarily carbohydrates and fat for energy. That "spares" protein the job of supplying large amounts of energy (except during exercise of unusual duration). But if carbohydrate intake drops too low, the body uses a significant quantity of protein for energy and less goes into developing muscles. The recipes that follow adhere to the proportion of carbohydrates (55-60 percent), fat (25-30 percent) and protein (15 percent) that you should include in your diet. The vegetarian dishes combine complementary proteins to assure a complete supply of amino acids.

Breakfast

. . . .

WHOLE-WHEAT HAZELNUT POPOVERS

All of the cholesterol in eggs is in the yolk. Using mostly whites, as you do in this recipe, provides protein and limits cholesterol.

Vegetable cooking spray	1/2 cup whole-wheat flour
1 cup lowfat milk (1% fat), approximately	1/2 cup unbleached white flour
1 egg	1/4 teaspoon salt
2 egg whites	2 tablespoons finely ground toasted hazelnuts

Preheat the oven to 400° F. Spray 10 popover pan cups or muffin tin cups with cooking spray. Place the pans in the oven to heat. Meanwhile, combine 1 cup of milk with the remaining ingredients in a blender and process just until smooth. Or, combine the ingredients in a medium-size bowl and whisk until smooth. Do not overblend or overbeat; the batter should be the consistency of heavy cream. Add 1 to 3 tablespoons more milk if necessary. Working quickly, fill the hot popover pans about 2/3 full; if using muffin tins, fill them almost to the top. Bake the popovers 20 minutes. Then, without opening the oven, reduce the temperature to 350° F and bake another 20 to 25 minutes. Remove the popovers from the pans and quickly prick the bottom of each one with a small sharp knife. Reduce the oven temperature to 200° F. Return the popovers to the oven to crisp for 15 minutes; they can be held in the oven for up to 40 minutes, if necessary. Serve warm.   Makes 10 large popovers

CALORIES per popover	75
56% Carbohydrate	11 g
19% Protein	4 g
25% Fat	2 g
CALCIUM	40 mg
IRON	.5 mg
SODIUM	84 mg

The nutritional analyses accompanying these recipes provide nutrient values per serving, unless otherwise indicated.

Whole-Wheat Hazelnut Popovers

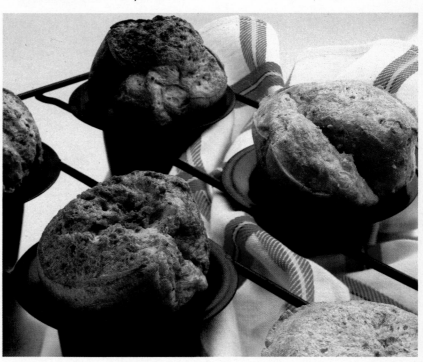

BUCKWHEAT-ALMOND PANCAKES WITH ORANGE-HONEY TOPPING

For high-quality protein, Glenn Town, director of the Exercise Physiology Lab at Wheaton College in Illinois, recommends combining grains like buckwheat with lowfat milk products, as this recipe does.

Vegetable cooking spray	1 egg, beaten
3/4 cup buckwheat flour	1 1/2 tablespoons safflower oil
3/4 cup whole-wheat flour	1/2 cup finely chopped toasted almonds
1 teaspoon baking powder	
1 teaspoon baking soda	1/2 cup orange juice
1/2 teaspoon salt	1/4 cup honey
1 1/4 cups buttermilk	

CALORIES	368
60% Carbohydrate	57 g
11% Protein	10 g
29% Fat	13 g
CALCIUM	191 mg
IRON	2 mg
SODIUM	689 mg

Spray a nonstick griddle or skillet with cooking spray and preheat it over medium-high heat. Combine the dry ingredients in a medium-size bowl. Add the buttermilk, egg, oil and 1/4 cup of water, and stir just to moisten the dry ingredients. Fold in the almonds. Using a scant 1/4 cup for each pancake, pour the batter onto the griddle or into the skillet. Cook the pancakes until the bubbles on the top burst and the edges appear dry. Turn the pancakes and cook until the undersides are golden. Transfer the pancakes to a platter and cover them with foil to keep warm. Repeat with the remaining batter. For the topping, warm the orange juice and honey in a small saucepan over low heat.

Makes twelve 4-inch pancakes (4 servings)

BUTTERMILK-SOY BISCUITS

The sunflower seeds in these biscuits are high in protein as well as fiber and vitamin A. Their high nutrient content makes the seeds alone a good post-workout snack.

Vegetable cooking spray	1/4 teaspoon salt
1 1/2 cups unbleached flour	3 tablespoons safflower oil
1/2 cup soy flour	3/4 cup plus 1 tablespoon buttermilk
2 teaspoons baking powder	1 tablespoon sunflower seeds
1 teaspoon baking soda	

Preheat the oven to 450° F. Lightly spray a large baking sheet with cooking spray. In a medium-size bowl stir together the dry ingredients using a fork. Add the oil and 3/4 cup of the buttermilk, and stir until a soft dough forms and leaves the sides of the bowl. Transfer the dough to a floured board and knead 8 times, then roll the dough out with a floured rolling pin to 1/2-inch thickness. Using a floured 2-inch biscuit cutter, cut the dough into 12 biscuits. Place the biscuits on the baking sheet, brush the tops with the remaining buttermilk and sprinkle with sunflower seeds. Bake on the middle rack of the oven 10 to 12 minutes, or until golden.

Makes 12 biscuits

CALORIES per biscuit	112
52% Carbohydrate	15 g
15% Protein	4 g
33% Fat	4 g
CALCIUM	71 mg
IRON	1 mg
SODIUM	204 mg

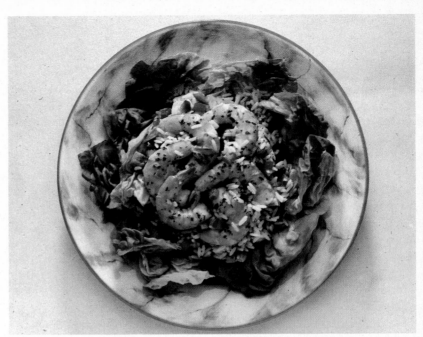

Spicy Shrimp Salad with Confetti Rice

Lunch

. . . .

CALORIES	326
41% Carbohydrate	33 g
31% Protein	25 g
28% Fat	10 g
CALCIUM	146 mg
IRON	5 mg
SODIUM	295 mg

SPICY SHRIMP SALAD WITH CONFETTI RICE

A 3 1/2-ounce serving of shrimp, a complete protein, has just one half the cholesterol of an egg yolk.

1 tablespoon pickling spice
1 1/4 pounds medium-size shrimp, in shells
3 tablespoons olive oil
2 garlic cloves, minced
1 teaspoon each dried, crushed basil, oregano and tarragon
1/4 teaspoon red pepper flakes

1/4 cup fresh lemon juice
1 tablespoon Dijon mustard
1/4 cup buttermilk
2 cups cooked white rice, cooled
1/2 cup finely chopped red bell pepper
1/2 cup chopped green bell pepper
1 head Boston lettuce
2 tablespoons finely chopped parsley

Stir the pickling spice into 1 quart of water in a medium-size saucepan and bring to a boil. Add the shrimp, cover, remove the pan from the heat, and let stand 6 to 8 minutes. Cool the shrimp in a colander under cold running water. Shell and devein the shrimp, reserving the shells. Transfer the shrimp to a medium-size bowl and set aside. Heat the oil in a medium-size skillet and add the shrimp shells, garlic, herbs and red pepper flakes. Cover and cook the mixture for 10 minutes, then strain it and add it to the shrimp. Combine the lemon juice, mustard and buttermilk in a small bowl, add the mixture to the shrimp and toss gently. Refrigerate the shrimp at least 2 hours, or overnight.

Combine the rice and peppers in a large bowl. Pour half of the sauce from the shrimp into the rice mixture; toss. Line a platter with lettuce and mound the rice on top. Arrange the shrimp on the rice and top with the remaining sauce. Sprinkle with chopped parsley. Makes 4 servings

TOFU SALAD WITH GINGER SAUCE

Research has shown that a diet high in soy-based foods such as tofu is associated with decreased blood cholesterol.

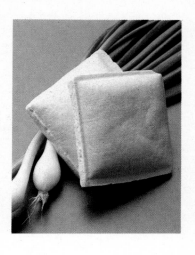

3 tablespoons reduced-sodium
   soy sauce
2 tablespoons balsamic or white
   wine vinegar
2 teaspoons Oriental sesame oil
1 1/2 tablespoons grated ginger
1 pound firm tofu (about 4
   blocks), drained, rinsed and cut
   into 3/4-inch cubes
3 cups shredded Romaine

1 cup alfalfa sprouts
2 cups cooked brown rice, cooled
8 cherry tomatoes
2 kirby cucumbers, peeled and diced
1 small red bell pepper, diced
1/4 pound white mushrooms, sliced
3 to 4 scallions, thinly sliced
1 tablespoon white sesame seeds,
   toasted

Stir together the soy sauce, vinegar, oil and ginger in a medium-size bowl. Add the tofu, stir gently and set aside to marinate at least 1 hour. Just before serving, divide the lettuce and sprouts among 4 plates and top with the marinated tofu. Divide the rice, tomatoes, cucumbers, peppers and mushrooms attractively among the plates and sprinkle with scallions and sesame seeds.

Makes 4 servings

CALORIES	280
51% Carbohydrate	37 g
21% Protein	15 g
28% Fat	9 g
CALCIUM	236 mg
IRON	5 mg
SODIUM	478 mg

THREE-BEAN CHILI

Eaten together, the beans and rice in this recipe provide complete protein. Each furnishes the essential amino acids the other lacks.

2/3 cup each canned pinto (pink)
   beans, black beans and red
   kidney beans
1/2 pound lean ground beef
1 cup coarsely chopped onion
1 garlic clove, chopped
1 1/2 cups coarsely chopped
   green bell pepper
1 cup sliced celery
2 teaspoons chili powder
1 teaspoon ground cumin

1/2 teaspoon ground oregano
2 cups coarsely chopped tomatoes
1/4 cup tomato paste
1 cup beef stock
1 teaspoon salt
2 cups hot cooked rice
Salsa (recipe on page 132)
1/2 cup coarsely chopped Spanish
   onion
1 cup shredded Cheddar cheese

Place the beans in a colander and rinse them well under cold running water; set them aside to drain. Heat a large nonstick saucepan over medium heat. Add the beef, onion and garlic to the pan and sauté until the beef is browned and the onion is translucent. Add 1 cup of the bell pepper and the celery, and continue cooking for 5 to 7 minutes, or until the vegetables begin to soften. Add the chili powder, cumin and oregano, and sauté for another minute. Add the tomatoes and tomato paste, the stock, the salt and the drained beans, reduce the heat to medium-low and simmer, partially covered, for 30 minutes. Divide the chili among 4 bowls and top each serving with 1/2 cup of rice and 1/2 cup of Salsa. Sprinkle each serving with the remaining 1/2 cup of bell pepper, the Spanish onion and the Cheddar cheese.   Makes 4 servings

CALORIES	572
49% Carbohydrate	72 g
21% Protein	31 g
30% Fat	19 g
CALCIUM	324 mg
IRON	7 mg
SODIUM	590 mg

CALORIES	54
79% Carbohydrate	12 g
14% Protein	2 g
7% Fat	.5 g
CALCIUM	34 mg
IRON	2 mg
SODIUM	80 mg

SALSA

3/4 pound ripe plum or cherry tomatoes, coarsely chopped

1 tablespoon finely chopped canned jalapeño peppers

1/2 cup chopped Spanish onion

2 tablespoons fresh lime juice

4 tablespoons fresh cilantro

Combine all the ingredients in a bowl. Let the salsa stand at room temperature for 30 to 45 minutes to allow the flavors to blend.   Makes 2 cups

CURRIED TURKEY SALAD

Turkey, one of the leanest types of poultry, has just as much protein as chicken and less fat. But stay away from "self-basting" birds; they are injected with butter or oil and are loaded with saturated fat.

1/2 cup mayonnaise-type salad dressing

1/2 cup plain lowfat yogurt

1/4 cup buttermilk

1/4 cup chopped chutney

1 1/2 teaspoons curry powder

1/8 teaspoon ground ginger

3 cups cooked turkey breast, cut into 1-inch cubes

13 1/4-ounce can juice-packed pineapple chunks, drained

1 cup thinly sliced celery

1/4 cup thinly sliced scallions

1/2 cup frozen green peas, thawed

1 Granny Smith or other tart green apple, peeled, cored and diced

Small head leaf lettuce

2 ounces snow peas, blanched

CALORIES	453
41% Carbohydrate	46 g
32% Protein	37 g
27% Fat	14 g
CALCIUM	161 mg
IRON	4 mg
SODIUM	404 mg

Combine the salad dressing, yogurt, buttermilk, chutney, curry powder and ginger in a small bowl; set aside. In a large bowl combine the turkey, pineapple, celery, scallions, peas and apple. Add the dressing and toss. Refrigerate the salad at least 2 hours. To serve, line a platter with lettuce and spoon the turkey salad on top. Garnish with snow peas.   Makes 4 servings

MISO CHICKEN SOUP WITH RICE NOODLES

Flavorful miso, a soy product, is high in protein and low in saturated fat .

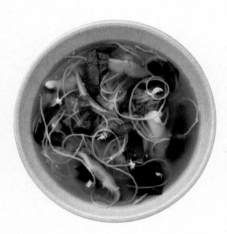

4 dried shiitake mushrooms, soaked 30 minutes in 1 cup warm water

4 cups low-sodium chicken stock

1 ounce dried rice noodles (mei fun) or spaghettini

1/4 cup miso

6 ounces skinless, boneless chicken breast, cut into thin strips

1/2 cup lightly packed spinach or bok choy leaves, torn into small pieces

1/8 teaspoon Oriental sesame oil

CALORIES	143
40% Carbohydrate	13 g
47% Protein	15 g
13% Fat	2 g
CALCIUM	33 mg
IRON	3 mg
SODIUM	91 mg

Strain the mushroom-soaking liquid into a medium-size saucepan. Add the stock and bring the mixture to a boil. Cut off and discard the mushroom stems. Slice the caps into slivers, add them to the stock along with the rice noodles and simmer for 3 to 4 minutes. Remove about 1/4 cup of stock and combine it with the miso in a small bowl; mix well and add to the soup. Add the chicken strips and bring the soup just to a boil. Add the spinach, remove the pan from the heat and stir in the sesame oil.   Makes 4 servings

Note: If shiitake mushrooms are unavailable, use 1/4 pound white mushrooms, thinly sliced, and add them with the rice noodles.

Dinner

CHICKEN SCALOPPINE WITH PEPPERS

When you remove the skin from chicken, you reduce the fat considerably and retain almost all of the protein.

CALORIES	205
17% Carbohydrate	9 g
55% Protein	29 g
28% Fat	6 g
CALCIUM	37 mg
IRON	2 mg
SODIUM	219 mg

1 lemon
4 skinless, boneless chicken
   breast halves (about 1 pound)
1/4 teaspoon salt
1/8 teaspoon freshly ground
   pepper
2 tablespoons flour

4 teaspoons vegetable oil
1 garlic clove, crushed
1 red and 1 yellow bell pepper, cut
   into 1/4-inch-wide strips
1/3 cup dry white wine
1/3 cup low-sodium chicken stock
1 tablespoon finely chopped parsley

Preheat the oven to 200° F. Halve the lemon and slice one half; reserve remaining half for juice. Cut the chicken breasts in half crosswise and pound gently to flatten them. Dry the chicken, sprinkle with salt, pepper and flour, and pat in the coating. Heat the oil and garlic in a large nonstick skillet over medium-high heat until the oil is hot; discard the garlic. Add a single layer of chicken pieces to the skillet, increase the heat to high and sauté for about 1 minute on each side, or until lightly browned. Keep the cooked chicken warm in the oven. Repeat for the remaining pieces. To the same skillet add the peppers, wine and 1 tablespoon of lemon juice and cook, covered, over medium-low heat for 5 minutes, or until the peppers are slightly softened. Uncover and cook over high heat another 5 minutes to reduce the liquid to about 2 tablespoons. Add the stock, bring to a boil and cook for 1 minute. Pour the sauce and peppers over the chicken, garnish with the lemon slices and sprinkle with parsley.   Makes 4 servings

Chicken Scaloppine with Peppers

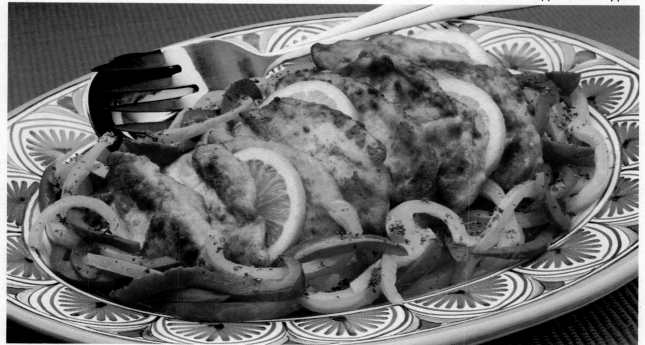

BAKED RED SNAPPER WITH GREEN SAUCE

CALORIES with sauce	180
8% Carbohydrate	4 g
64% Protein	27 g
28% Fat	5 g
CALCIUM	54 mg
IRON	1 mg
SODIUM	108 mg

The polyunsaturated fats in red snapper and other fish are good for your heart and blood vessels. As well as lowering blood cholesterol, they contain eicosapentaenoic acid (EPA), which has been associated with reduced blood fats and lowered blood pressure.

2- to 2 1/2-pound whole red snapper, cleaned, head and tail left on
2 tablespoons lemon juice

2 teaspoons olive oil
Parsley sprigs for garnish
Green Sauce (see following recipe)

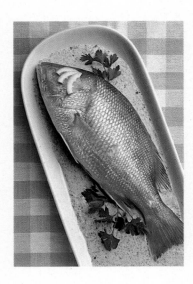

Preheat the oven to 400° F. Rinse and dry the fish. Rub the inside and outside of the fish with lemon juice, and oil the outside. Place the fish in an ovenproof serving dish or on a large piece of foil in a baking pan. Bake for 20 to 25 minutes, or until the fish just begins to exude juices and the cavity is no longer pink. Transfer the fish to a warm serving platter if necessary, garnish with parsley sprigs and serve with Green Sauce.   Makes 4 servings

GREEN SAUCE

1 1/2 teaspoons olive oil
1/2 teaspoon minced garlic
1/3 cup dry white wine
1/2 cup fish stock or chicken stock

1/4 cup plain lowfat yogurt mixed with
1 1/2 teaspoons arrowroot
1/8 teaspoon white pepper
3 tablespoons minced fresh parsley

Heat the oil in a small saucepan over medium heat. Add the garlic and sauté over low heat until golden. Add the wine, increase the heat to high and cook for about 10 minutes, or until reduced by half. Add the stock and bring to a boil. Whisk in the yogurt mixture and the pepper, and stir until the sauce comes to a boil. Remove the sauce from the heat and stir in the parsley. Serve hot.   Makes 4 servings

COLD NOODLES AND CHICKEN WITH SESAME SAUCE

Oriental sesame oil and sesame paste, now available in many supermarkets, are so flavorful you can use very little of each in this lowfat version of a Chinese restaurant favorite.

CALORIES	511
41% Carbohydrate	52 g
29% Protein	37 g
30% Fat	17 g
CALCIUM	109 mg
IRON	4 mg
SODIUM	394 mg

1/2 pound angel hair pasta
1 tablespoon Oriental sesame oil
1/4 cup sesame paste (tahini)
1 garlic clove, peeled and crushed
1 teaspoon sugar
2 tablespoons reduced-sodium soy sauce
3 tablespoons balsamic or red wine vinegar

1/2 teaspoon hot pepper sauce
1 cup low-sodium chicken stock, approximately
1/2 pound skinless cooked chicken breast, shredded
1 medium-size cucumber, peeled and cut into thin strips
2 tablespoons unsalted dry-roasted peanuts, chopped
1/4 cup thinly sliced scallions

Cook the pasta according to the package directions. Drain the pasta in a colander, cool under cold water and drain. Return the pasta to the pot and toss it with the sesame oil. Combine the sesame paste, garlic, sugar, soy sauce, vinegar and hot pepper sauce in a blender and process, adding enough chicken stock to make a smooth sauce. Place the chicken in a large bowl, add half of the sauce and toss gently. Mix the remaining sauce with the pasta and toss gently with your hands to separate the strands. Transfer the pasta to a shallow serving bowl, top with the cucumber strips, then with the chicken, and sprinkle with the peanuts and scallions.   Makes 4 servings

BRAISED RABBIT WITH MUSTARD SAUCE

Rabbit, often overlooked as a lowfat protein source, looks and tastes like chicken when cooked.

2 1/2-pound rabbit, skinned and
   cut into 6 pieces, liver reserved
1/4 cup all-purpose flour
2 tablespoons vegetable oil
1/4 teaspoon salt
1/8 teaspoon black pepper
1 tablespoon minced fresh thyme
   or 1 teaspoon dried thyme
1/2 cup each finely chopped
   carrots, celery and onion

1 garlic clove, minced
1/2 cup dry white wine
1/2 cup low-sodium chicken stock
1 cup plain lowfat yogurt
1 tablespoon arrowroot
2 tablespoons whole-grain Dijon
   mustard
1 tablespoon finely chopped fresh
   parsley for garnish

Preheat the oven to 350° F. Finely chop the liver; set aside. Dry the rabbit pieces and dredge with flour; shake off the excess. Heat the oil in a large ovenproof skillet. Add the rabbit pieces and cook over high heat for about 5 minutes, or until brown on both sides. Sprinkle with the salt, pepper and thyme, and cook for another 2 minutes. Remove the rabbit pieces to a platter; pour off all but 1 tablespoon of fat from the skillet. Add the liver, carrots, celery, onion and garlic, and cook over medium heat, stirring and mashing the liver with a spoon. When the vegetables are softened and the liver is no longer pink, add the wine and stir to incorporate any browned bits clinging to the bottom. Cook, stirring, until the wine is reduced by half. Add the stock and bring to a simmer. Return the rabbit to the skillet, cover tightly and braise in the oven 20 to 25 minutes, or until tender.

Meanwhile, combine the yogurt, arrowroot and mustard in a small bowl and mix well. When the rabbit is done, transfer to a serving platter and keep warm. Strain the braising liquid and return it to the skillet; reheat the liquid and whisk in the yogurt mixture. Cook over medium heat until hot; do not boil. Pour the sauce over the rabbit and sprinkle with parsley.   Makes 4 servings

CALORIES	327
23% Carbohydrate	18 g
43% Protein	34 g
34% Fat	12 g
CALCIUM	161 mg
IRON	3 mg
SODIUM	486 mg

CORNMEAL-CRUST PIZZA WITH MUSHROOM SAUCE

During week-long races, competitive cyclists eat high-protein, high-calcium dishes like this one for their evening recovery meals.

CALORIES		376
	49% Carbohydrate	49 g
	18% Protein	17 g
	33% Fat	13 g
CALCIUM		361 mg
IRON		3 mg
SODIUM		175 mg

1 1/2 cups stone-ground cornmeal
1/4 cup grated Parmesan cheese
2 teaspoons olive oil
1 medium-size onion, peeled and finely chopped
1 garlic clove, crushed

3/4 pound fresh white mushrooms, trimmed and thinly sliced
1 cup canned crushed tomatoes
1/4 teaspoon dried oregano, crumbled
1/4 teaspoon dried basil, crumbled
1/8 teaspoon red pepper flakes
1 cup shredded Swiss cheese

For the crust, bring 3 1/2 cups of water to a boil in a large saucepan. Meanwhile, mix 1 cup of cold water with the cornmeal to make a thick paste. Stir the cornmeal mixture into the boiling water and cook, stirring constantly, for 10 to 12 minutes, or until thick and smooth. Remove the pan from the heat, stir in the Parmesan, and mix well. Spread the mixture evenly in a nonstick 12" pizza pan or spread it in a 12" round on a large baking sheet, smoothing it with a spatula. Let the crust stand at room temperature at least 1 hour, or until thoroughly cool and dry on the surface.

Preheat the oven to 350° F. Bake the crust 45 minutes. Meanwhile, for the sauce, heat the oil in a large nonstick skillet and add the onion, garlic and mushrooms. Cook, stirring, until any liquid evaporates and the mushrooms are lightly browned. Add the tomatoes, herbs and pepper flakes and cook over low heat, stirring occasionally, another 5 minutes. Spread the sauce over the crust, top with the Swiss cheese and bake about 5 minutes, or until bubbly and hot.   Makes 4 servings

MANHATTAN FISH CHOWDER

Potatoes do not include all of the essential amino acids. But when you eat them with a complete animal protein like fish, your body gets full use of the seven essential amino acids potatoes do contain.

2 tablespoons olive oil
1 cup finely chopped onion
1 garlic clove, peeled and crushed
1 1/2 cups peeled, diced potatoes
1 1/2 cups fish stock plus 1 1/2 cups low-sodium chicken stock, or 3 cups chicken stock

Small bay leaf
1/2 teaspoon salt
1 cup canned crushed tomatoes
1/4 teaspoon dried thyme
1/4 teaspoon crushed fennel seed
1/4 teaspoon red pepper flakes
1 pound skinless, boneless halibut, cut into 1-inch chunks
1/4 cup finely chopped parsley

CALORIES		264
	26% Carbohydrate	16 g
	44% Protein	27 g
	30% Fat	8 g
CALCIUM		57 mg
IRON		3 mg
SODIUM		479 mg

Heat the oil in a large saucepan. Add the onion and garlic and cook over medium heat until softened. Add the potatoes, stock, bay leaf and salt, cover the pan, and bring to a simmer. Cook for about 15 minutes, or until the potatoes are tender. Add the remaining ingredients except the parsley, bring just to a boil and stir gently. Remove the pan from the heat, sprinkle the chowder with parsley and serve.   Makes 4 servings

Desserts

HAZELNUT CHEESECAKE

*Most cheesecakes are loaded with fat and cholesterol. This recipe cuts back
on the fat by using lowfat milk products and just one egg yolk.*

Vegetable cooking spray

3 ounces shelled, roasted, hulled
   hazelnuts, finely ground

1 pound skim-milk ricotta cheese

2 cups lowfat lemon yogurt

1 egg

1 egg white

1/4 cup arrowroot

2/3 cup sugar

1/2 teaspoon vanilla extract

1/4 teaspoon almond extract

1/4 teaspoon salt

1/4 teaspoon grated lemon peel

CALORIES	237
48% Carbohydrate	29 g
15% Protein	9 g
37% Fat	10 g
CALCIUM	212 mg
IRON	.6 mg
SODIUM	150 mg

Preheat the oven to 300° F. Lightly coat a 7-inch springform pan with cooking
spray. Reserving 1 tablespoon of ground hazelnuts, combine all of the remaining ingredients in a medium-size bowl and mix well. Pour the mixture into the
pan and bake for 1 hour. Turn off the oven and let the cake cool in the
unopened oven for 1 1/2 to 2 hours, then cool the cake at room temperature
for another 1 1/2 hours. Remove the cake from the pan and sprinkle the top
with the reserved ground hazelnuts. Refrigerate the cake for 3 to 4 hours, or
overnight, before serving.   Makes 10 servings

Hazelnut Cheesecake

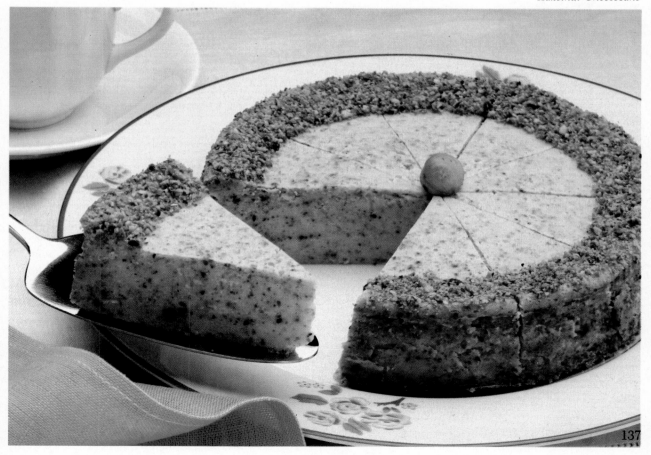

RICE PUDDING WITH STRAWBERRY SAUCE

When you eat milk and rice together, the complete protein in milk enables your body to make better use of the incomplete protein in rice.

4 cups lowfat milk (1% fat)	1/2 cup plus 1 tablespoon sugar
1/2 cup long-grain white rice	2 teaspoons vanilla extract
1/8 teaspoon salt	1 cup evaporated skim milk
1/4 cup raisins	1/2 teaspoon cinnamon
2 eggs	1 pint strawberries, hulled and sliced
1 egg white	2 tablespoons orange juice

Preheat the oven to 350° F. Combine the milk, rice and salt in a large saucepan, bring to a simmer and cook for 30 minutes. Add the raisins and simmer the rice for another 5 to 10 minutes, or until thick but not dry. Remove the pan from the heat. Beat together the eggs, egg white, 1/2 cup of the sugar, vanilla and milk in a large bowl. Stir 1/3 cup of the rice into the egg mixture, then add this to the saucepan and stir to combine. Pour the mixture into an 8 x 8" glass baking dish and set the dish in a larger pan on the middle oven rack. Pour 1" of hot water into the larger pan. Sprinkle the pudding with cinnamon. Bake 25 to 30 minutes, or until the pudding is loosely set but still quivers when shaken. Remove the pudding from the hot-water bath and chill if desired.

For the strawberry sauce, purée the berries with the remaining sugar and the orange juice in a blender. To serve, spoon the pudding onto dessert plates and top with sauce.   Makes 8 servings

CALORIES	228
71% Carbohydrate	41 g
17% Protein	10 g
12% Fat	3 g
CALCIUM	263 mg
IRON	1 mg
SODIUM	158 mg

SWEET YOGURT CHEESE WITH BERRIES

Yogurt cheese is an excellent substitute for cream cheese, sour cream or whipped cream. It is low in fat and salt and high in protein and calcium.

2 cups Yogurt Cheese (recipe follows)	1/4 teaspoon each ground nutmeg and cardamom
1/4 teaspoon vanilla extract	2 teaspoons raspberry jam
2 tablespoons honey	1 pint fresh raspberries, washed

Place the Yogurt Cheese, vanilla extract, honey and spices in a small bowl and mix well. Lightly stir in the jam; do not overmix. Line a small bowl with a long sheet of plastic wrap, spoon in the yogurt mixture and overlap the ends of the plastic wrap on top. Refrigerate for 2 to 3 hours. Unmold the chilled cheese onto a platter and arrange the berries around it.   Makes 6 servings

CALORIES	128
59% Carbohydrate	20 g
24% Protein	8 g
17% Fat	3 g
CALCIUM	219 mg
IRON	.4 mg
SODIUM	75 mg

YOGURT CHEESE

1 quart plain lowfat yogurt

Line a large colander with several thicknesses of cheesecloth and set it over a deep bowl. Pour in the yogurt, cover with plastic wrap, and place a small plate and a weight on top. Let stand 3 to 4 hours, or until the yogurt is the consistency of soft cream cheese.   Makes about 2 cups

CALORIES per 1/4 cup	59
37% Carbohydrate	5 g
37% Protein	6 g
26% Fat	2 g
CALCIUM	156 mg
IRON	.05 mg
SODIUM	56 mg

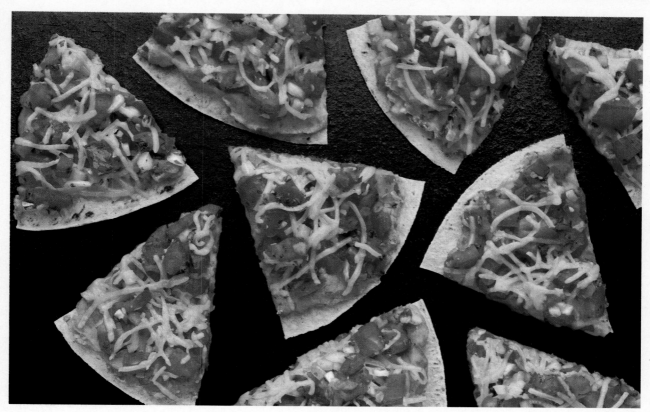

Nachos

Snacks
. . . .

NACHOS

Corn tortillas and beans are complementary proteins as well as good sources of complex carbohydrates.

CALORIES	144
50% Carbohydrate	19 g
20% Protein	7 g
30% Fat	5 g
CALCIUM	166 mg
IRON	2 mg
SODIUM	251 mg

Eight 6-inch corn tortillas
1 1/4 cups kidney beans,
    drained, liquid reserved

1/4 teaspoon chili powder
2 cups Salsa (see page 132), drained
1 cup shredded Monterey Jack cheese

Preheat the oven to 500° F. Immerse the tortillas one at a time in water; drain and lay them on baking sheets. Bake tortillas for 6 or 7 minutes, or just until crisp, turning them after 4 to 5 minutes. If the tortillas begin to curl, lay another baking sheet on top of them. Remove the tortillas from the baking sheet, using a metal spatula to loosen them if necessary, and set aside to cool. Reduce the oven temperature to 350° F.

Combine the beans and chili powder in a small skillet and heat over medium heat, mashing the beans with a fork, until the mixture is hot. Stir in the reserved bean liquid a little at a time until the mixture is smooth and spreadable. Cut each tortilla into 6 wedges, then reassemble the wedges into rounds on the baking sheet. Spread the bean mixture equally over the tortillas and top each with 1/4 cup of Salsa and 2 tablespoons of cheese. Layer on the remaining Salsa and cheese. Bake for 4 to 5 minutes, or until the cheese is melted. Serve hot.

Makes 8 servings

SARDINE CANAPES

Rich in protein, sardines are also high in calcium when eaten with the bones.

CALORIES per canapé	34
44% Carbohydrate	4 g
26% Protein	2 g
30% Fat	1 g
CALCIUM	24 mg
IRON	.3 mg
SODIUM	105 mg

Two 2 3/4-ounce cans sardines in oil, drained
1 hard-boiled egg
1 teaspoon capers, drained
2 teaspoons lemon juice
1 tablespoon Dijon-style mustard
1/8 teaspoon hot pepper sauce
1/4 cup finely chopped celery
1/4 cup finely chopped fresh dill
28 melba toast rounds

Place the sardines in a food processor or blender and process briefly. Blend in the remaining ingredients, except the toast rounds, one by one, pushing the mixture down with a rubber spatula after each addition. Refrigerate the mixture at least 2 hours, or until well chilled. Spread each piece of melba toast with 1 tablespoon of the sardine mixture.

Makes 28 canapés

SPICY CHEESE SPREAD

This savory snack cheese, unlike most cheese spreads, is made with lowfat milk products.

CALORIES	68
39% Carbohydrate	7 g
41% Protein	7 g
20% Fat	2 g
CALCIUM	52 mg
IRON	.4 mg
SODIUM	108 mg

1 pound dry curd cottage cheese
1 cup Yogurt Cheese (see page 138)
1 tablespoon Dijon mustard
1 teaspoon caraway seeds, crushed
2 tablespoons sweet or hot paprika
3 tablespoons finely chopped chives
32 plain crackers

Place all of the ingredients except the crackers in a medium-size bowl and mix well. Cover and refrigerate at least 2 hours, or overnight, to allow the flavors to blend. Spread each cracker with 1 tablespoon of cheese spread.

Makes 16 servings

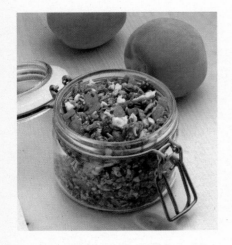

GRANOLA

The rolled oats in granola contain cholesterol-lowering fiber. And, calorie for calorie, oats contain twice as much protein as wheat does.

CALORIES per 1/4 cup	124
60% Carbohydrate	20 g
10% Protein	3 g
30% Fat	4 g
CALCIUM	26 mg
IRON	1 mg
SODIUM	4 mg

3 cups rolled oats
1/2 cup sunflower seeds
3 tablespoons sesame seeds
1/4 cup wheat germ
1/4 teaspoon cinnamon
1/4 cup honey
6 tablespoons safflower oil
3/4 cup chopped dried apples
3/4 cup golden raisins

Preheat the oven to 350° F. Combine the oats, sunflower seeds, sesame seeds, wheat germ and cinnamon in a large bowl. Stir together the honey and oil, pour over the oat mixture and toss to coat the dry ingredients. Spread the mixture in two shallow 9 x 13" baking pans and bake on the middle rack of the oven 15 minutes, stirring frequently. Allow the granola to cool. Stir the dried fruit into the cooled granola. Store in a covered container in the refrigerator.

Makes about 5 1/2 cups

Beverages

BUTTERMILK COOLER

Wherever possible, substitute buttermilk for whole milk in your meals. Buttermilk has the same amount of protein as whole milk but 75 percent less fat. This cooler makes a delicious breakfast drink or a satisfying snack.

1 cup buttermilk	1 cup sliced fresh strawberries or 1 cup unsweetened frozen strawberries
1 egg	
1 tablespoon honey	
	Seltzer or club soda (optional)

Combine the buttermilk, egg, honey and strawberries in a blender and process until smooth and creamy. Add seltzer for a lighter drink, or to stretch the drink to 2 servings.   Makes 1 large serving

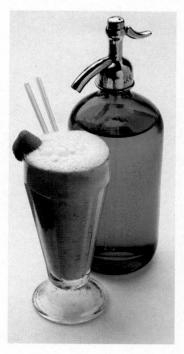

CALORIES	287
55% Carbohydrate	40 g
20% Protein	15 g
25% Fat	8 g
CALCIUM	335 mg
IRON	2 mg
SODIUM	329 mg

ZESTY TOMATO DRINK

The vitamin C from the tomato juice in this drink helps your body absorb the iron from the beef stock.

1 cup tomato juice	2 tablespoons plain lowfat yogurt
1/2 cup beef stock	Lemon wedge for garnish
1/4 cup peeled and coarsely chopped tomato	

Combine the tomato juice, beef stock, tomato and yogurt in a blender and process until smooth. Serve over ice, garnished with a lemon wedge.

Makes 1 serving

Note: If you wish, flavor this drink with herbs such as basil, dill or oregano, or for a spicy drink add a dash of hot pepper sauce.

CALORIES	77
72% Carbohydrate	16 g
18% Protein	4 g
10% Fat	1 g
CALCIUM	77 mg
IRON	2 mg
SODIUM	907 mg

SPICED YOGURT SHAKE

Milkshakes are high in protein and calcium, but they are also full of butterfat. This drink supplies just as much calcium and protein as the average milkshake and does so without the saturated fat. This drink is based on an Indian beverage, lassi.

1 1/2 cups plain lowfat yogurt	1/2 teaspoon ground cardamom
1/2 cup lowfat milk (1% fat)	1/2 teaspoon cinnamon
2 tablespoons honey	1/4 teaspoon ground coriander

Combine the yogurt, milk, honey and spices in a blender and process until smooth and creamy.   Makes 2 servings

CALORIES	200
64% Carbohydrate	33 g
21% Protein	11 g
15% Fat	3 g
CALCIUM	397 mg
IRON	.5 mg
SODIUM	151 mg

PROP CREDITS

Cover: sweat pants–The Gap, San Francisco, Calif.; page 6: leotard–Dance France LTD., Santa Monica, Calif; pages 26-27: dumbbells, ankle and wrist weights–Triangle, Morrisville, N.C.; mat, lifters–Excel, Pico Rivera, Calif.; weight bar–Gemfitness, New York City; pages 28-29: see pages listed for individual exercises; page 30: shirt, shorts–Naturalife, New York City; pages 36-53: leotard–Marika, San Diego, Calif.; mat–Gemfitness, New York City; weight bench–Fitness Depot, New York City; ankle weight–Triangle, Morrisville, N.C.; shoes–Nautilus Athletic Footwear, Inc., Greenville, S.C.; pages 60-93: leotard, tights–Dance France LTD., Santa Monica, Calif.; shorts–Sportco, Beaverton, Ore.; mat–Triangle, Morrisville, N.C.; page 94: sweat pants–Naturalife, New York City; pages 100-123: tights–Danskin, Inc., New York City; shoes–Avia, Inc., Portland, Ore.; Nautilus Athletic Footwear, Greenville, S.C.; weights, lifters–Gemfitness, New York City; weight bench–Fitness Depot, New York City; page 124: ceramic bowl–Broadway Panhandler, New York City; Calphalon saucepan–Commercial Aluminum Cookware Co., Toledo, Ohio; page 130: plate–Ad Hoc Housewares, New York City; page 133: platter–Ceramica Mia South, New York City; serving utensils–Broadway Panhandler, New York City; page 139: plate, cake server–Gear, New York City; page 141: seltzer bottle–Gimme Seltzer, New York City.

ACKNOWLEDGMENTS

All cosmetics and grooming products supplied by Clinique Labs, Inc., New York City

Off-camera warm-up equipment: rowing machine supplied by Precor USA, Redmond, Wash.; Tunturi stationary bicycle supplied by Amerec Corp., Bellevue, Wash.

Washing machine and dryer supplied by White-Westinghouse, Columbus, Ohio

Index prepared by Ian Tucker

Production by Giga Communications

PHOTOGRAPHY CREDIT

All photographs by Steven Mays, Rebus, Inc.

ILLUSTRATION CREDITS

Page 8, illustration: David Flaherty; page 10, illustration: Brian Sisco; page 11, illustration: David Flaherty; page 13, illustration: David Flaherty; page 14, illustration: David Flaherty; page 19, illustration: Durell Godfrey; pages 20-21, illustrations: Dana Burns; page 25, illustrations: Durell Godfrey; page 33, illustration: Dana Burns; pages 34-35, illustrations: Durell Godfrey; page 57, illustration: Dana Burns; page 59, illustrations, Durell Godfrey; page 97, illustration: Dana Burns; pages 98-99, illustrations: Durell Godfrey.

Time-Life Books Inc. offers a wide range of fine recordings, including a Big Band series. For subscription information, call 1-800-621-7026, or write TIME-LIFE MUSIC, Time & Life Building, Chicago, Illinois 60611.

INDEX

Abdominal-hold test, 19
abdominal muscles, 55-57
    exercises for, 60-75
    warm-ups for, 58-59
abductors, 33
    exercises for, 44-47
Achilles tendon, 33
aerobic endurance, 10, 16-17
amino acids, 126
ankle weights, 26, 27
arm muscles, 95-97
    exercises for, 100-117, 121-123
ATP (adenosine triphosphate), 14

Back muscles (lower), 56
    exercises for, 76-93
back muscles (upper), 95-97
    exercises for, 100-113, 120-123
    warm-ups for, 98-99
back problems, 10, 13, 17, 64, 76, 79
bar lifts, 118-121
bench flys, 97, 110
bench presses, 97, 110
bent-arm hang, 97, 123
beverage recipes, 141
biceps, 95-97
    exercises for, 110, 112-114, 116,
        121-123
bicycle exercise, 70-71
body assessment, 18
body type, 12, 18
bone loss, 9
breakfast recipes, 128-129
breathing, 23, 57

Calcium
    amounts in recipe dishes, 128-141
    recommended dietary intake of, 127
calf muscles, 33
    exercises for, 52-53
calories, 127-141
    amounts in recipe dishes, 128-141
carbohydrates
    amounts in recipe dishes, 128-141
    recommended dietary intake of, 127
cardiovascular endurance, 10, 16-17
cellulite, 32
chest muscles, 95-97
    exercises for, 100-111, 119, 120
    warm-ups for, 98-99
chinning (chin-ups), 97, 122-123
cholesterol, 126-127
cool-down, 23
CP (creatine phosphate), 14
crunches, 15, 57, 60-66

Dehydration, 15
deltoids, 95-97
    exercises for, 100-109, 114, 115,
        118-120
dessert recipes, 137-138
dinner recipes, 133-136
dips, 97, 108-109
dumbbells, 26, 27

Endurance, 9, 10, 16
energy for building muscles, 14
equipment, 26-27
erector spinae, 56
    exercises for, 76-93
essential amino acids, 126
exercise mats, 26, 27
external obliques, 56
    exercises for, 62-64, 70-71

Fat, body
    abdominal, 56
    loss of, 13, 15
    vs. muscle, 10, 12-13, 15
    pinch test for, 18
    on thighs and hips, 31-32
fat, dietary, 126-141
    amounts in recipe dishes, 128-141
    recommended dietary intake of, 127
fitness assessment, 16-17
flexibility, 9, 13

Gastrocnemius, 33
gluteus maximus, 32
    exercises for, 40-43
gluteus medius, 33
    exercises for, 44-47

Hamstrings, 32-33
    exercises for, 40-43
hip flexors, 32, 60, 79
hips
    body fat on, 31-32
    exercises for, 45-51
    muscles of, 32, 33

Internal obliques, 56
    exercises for, 62-64, 70-71
iron
    amounts in recipe dishes, 128-141
    recommended dietary intake of, 127

Joint flexibility, 9, 13

Lactic acid, 14
latissimus dorsi, 95-97
    exercises for, 100-113, 121-123
leg exercises, see lower body exercises
lifters, 26, 27
lower body exercises, 31-53
    gluteal work, 40-43
    hamstring work, 40-43
    inner-thigh work, 49-51
    lower body muscles, 31-33
    lower-leg work, 52-53
    outer-thigh work, 44-48
    quadriceps work, 36-39
lunch recipes, 130-132

Mental functioning and exercise, 9
middle body exercises, 55-75
    abdominal work, 60-75
    back work, 76-93
    middle body muscles, 55-57
    warm-ups, 58-59
motivation, 12
muscle balance, 22
muscles
    vs. body fat, 10, 12-13, 15
    energy for, 14
    exercises for, see muscle shaping and
        toning exercises
    growth of, 11
    loss of, 17
    of lower body, 31-33
    major groups of, 20-21
    of middle body, 55-57
    soreness of, 24
    of upper body, 95-97
muscle shaping and toning exercises, 7-29
    aerobic endurance and, 10
    back problems and, 10, 13, 17, 64, 76, 79
    basic workout, 28-29
    benefits of, 9-10
    body assessment, 18
    body fat loss and, 13, 15
    choosing, 20
    common mistakes with, 24-25
    equipment for, 26-27
    fitness assessment and, 16
    flexibility and, 9, 13
    guidelines for working out, 23
    for lower body see lower body
        exercises
    motivation and, 12
    protein consumption and, 15
    strength tests, 19
    vs. swimming, 10
    training keys, 22
    training regimen, 10-12, 22